Madhouse

Madhouse

PJ GALLAGHER

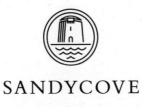

SANDYCOVE

an imprint of

PENGUIN BOOKS

SANDYCOVE

UK | USA | Canada | Ireland | Australia
India | New Zealand | South Africa

Sandycove is part of the Penguin Random House group of companies
whose addresses can be found at global.penguinrandomhouse.com.

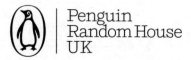

First published 2023

001

Set in 13.5/16pt Garamond MT Std
Typeset by Jouve (UK), Milton Keynes
Printed and bound in Great Britain by Clays Ltd, Elcograf S.p.A.

The authorized representative in the EEA is Penguin Random House Ireland,
Morrison Chambers, 32 Nassau Street, Dublin D02 YH68

A CIP catalogue record for this book is available from the British Library

ISBN: 978–1–844–88597–8

www.greenpenguin.co.uk

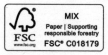

This book is dedicated to Stevie and Milo.
Where this book finishes, your story begins.

Contents

CONTENTS

Introduction

Whack-a-mole

July 2021

When I was a youngster, I remember thinking, 'Oh, my God, our family's mental, but one day, maybe I'll be a part of a different family.'

Then that developed into: 'I never want to be a part of any family ever because all families are nuts.'

But then I look at my sister and she's the exact flip, the complete opposite to me. She's got three kids and she's married. Marriage is hard work no matter who you are, but she does a good job. She's functional, a member of society.

Stacey does worry about things but here's what she worries about: 'My kids, are they well? What are we going to do for them? I've a few problems at work, how do I solve them? My husband, I hope he's all right.'

My worries are more along the line of, 'How am I not going to be homeless next week? How am I going to stop myself from being murdered by the end of next month?'

It's just off the rails. Catastrophic. A lot of my time is spent walking around looking for disaster in normal situations.

That's my hobby, wondering when the next terrible thing is going to happen, imagining every possible outcome of every decision until it ends badly in my head.

Since the very start I've been thinking the worst is going to happen, but in my own defence, I was born and I was given away. Then I went somewhere else, until at six months of age I ended up with Sean and Helen Gallagher in the northside of Dublin. When I was nine, six people with severe long-term psychiatric issues came to live in our house. So, mad things did keep happening, the blueprint is there.

Now, I look at Stacey and I think: 'How in the name of God have you got to a place in your life where you don't think crazy things are going to happen? How do you do it? How do you get to a place in your head where you think to yourself: *Things will be okay, tomorrow will be just like today*?'

Because I would say for a huge part of our lives, tomorrow was never okay. Tomorrow was always something to be genuinely very worried about. Coming home from school and there's an ambulance outside the gaff and you don't know who is getting into it. Home was a place where anything could and did happen. I wasn't even ten years old and everything had happened. Everything. The emotions I had then are the emotions I still have today but now, at forty-six, I'm running out of potential. I'm rapidly running out of potential.

At least when you're a kid there's an element of you that thinks *anything is possible*. You think, 'Okay, maybe I can't play for Dublin, but, hey, maybe I will become an astronaut, maybe I will become the president. Maybe I will.' You have those fantasies.

Now, I look in the mirror and I see an old man looking back, and I think, 'Maybe you will have your own hip until you're seventy.' It's a different aspiration.

Your forties is the stage of your life where you want stability, but looking in the mirror I feel less secure than I've ever felt in my life. That's why part of me is saying that I have to tell the truth about everything in this book, because I've always slapped everything down, been playing whack-a-mole my whole life. Just hiding the problems, not trying to eradicate the moles, just pushing them back into their holes for a bit.

There's so many moles now. Maybe I had ten moles when I was young, but I have at least sixty now and I have to just turn around and be honest and say, 'Look, I can't control these moles, I can't control any of them.'

February 2023

At the time I was writing about those sixty moles in the summer of 2021 I really thought I was in control of my life; I was writing a book, working on the radio, in a long-term relationship.

Only a few weeks later I was doing that thing I always do, catastrophizing about the book, about a potential fallout with my mother or, worse still, about humiliating her and embarrassing myself. What I wanted to do was tell the truth, but I decided I couldn't, and I stepped away from the book altogether. By December I was off the wall, completely sick, with zero control over anything.

Coming to the realization I couldn't write this book was probably the beginning of me getting very, very ill but not recognizing it. It really is that slow and steady a slide into a bad place.

Less than six months after I wrote about those sixty moles they clubbed together and became one big shady panic mole. He's the fellow that chased me into St Patrick's Hospital. He's the bollox that tried to kill me.

When I first went into the hospital, they asked me to come up with a name for my illness so that it would feel separate to myself. The name I came up with is Patrick. But Patrick is my name and that's my problem pretty much in a nutshell: I came up with a name to describe my illness that was actually my own name. The counsellor was like: 'This is ridiculous: you've called your panic Patrick, your depression Paddy and you're PJ?'

They were the only names I could think of.

Now I know what I should have called my illness: Noel the Big Bastard Mole.

As I'm writing this it's a year since I left St Pat's. When I got out I thought I was never going to have a bad day again, I thought: 'No matter what, I've defeated that mole, he's gone down like a bouncy castle, he's not getting me.'

Now, of course, life is kicking in. Now I have to get a divorce. On the 13th of May 2023 I'll have been married for ten years and separated for eight of them. But not, of course, properly separated, because, God forbid I'd do it the right way. God forbid I'd go and talk to a solicitor or get anything on paper. No, no, just ignore it, it'll be grand, stay married forever.

As well as that I'm waiting for two babies to arrive with my partner Kelly and that's a whole new bag of moles right there. Most people would have one baby but, of course, I'm having two.

But at least I know I'm not sick, I just have a tragic case of idiocy, and that's all right, I can manage that. That was always the way.

When I first started writing this book my main worry was my ma and how she would take it. I talked to my sister Stacey about what I would and wouldn't say. She thought telling the truth about how we grew up was a good idea, that children grow up around addiction and it's important to talk about it.

But at the time my ma was still alive. It was during the pandemic and I was living with her and really worried about hurting her feelings and embarrassing her. I was also afraid of bringing it up with her, of the confrontation that would entail because even though I'm in my late forties I've always felt like an eleven-year-old whenever my ma was upset with me.

The other problem is I always tried to hide everything from my mother. It was cover up, cover up, cover up. I always tried to cover up everything.

You know when you're younger and there's like a lad and he calls his parents by their first names – have you ever known one of them? An eleven-year-old who calls his father 'Brendan'? Looks at his mother and says, 'How are you, Jane, how are you doing today?' Kids who drink a glass of wine with their parents at dinner when they're sixteen. Or they get a tasteful tattoo on their back after much family deliberation.

It wasn't like that in our house. Years ago, when I got my first tattoo, I was doing a sketch with Jason Byrne and I made him put his hand over it in case word got back to my ma. She always said tattoos were only for mad men and 'huers'. I hid smoking and drinking and girlfriends from her because around her, I always felt I wasn't old enough to be doing anything. I hid everything. Up to the point that until the day she died I would still cover my arms up so my ma couldn't see the hundreds of tattoos I have drawn all over them. As if she didn't know.

And what did it matter if she did? It's not like I was suddenly going to try and apply for a job in a bank. At this stage, it wouldn't matter if I had a tattoo of a balaclava on my face.

But there was just no way I could tell this story honestly without discussing the drinking. How could I leave out the booze? Booze was the main problem in our house and was the context for everything. Booze was the wobbly rock the whole thing was founded on. Without it there's no real explanation for anything else. Without it the book would just be a series of anecdotes that don't really tell you *why* anything happened because it would take two main players off the table: my folks.

All that would be left would be an article, like those ones you read about some ex-squaddie who gets turned into a hippy after he takes a load of ayahuasca. You read it and you think, *This is just about a very boring man who found drugs and likes sitting in the woods.* It doesn't really explain anything.

When we made the play *Madhouse*, about my childhood, my ma came to see it. But that was safe because it was a comedy about a young boy growing up in unusual circumstances and we didn't go too much into the darker stuff. No one in that play was drunk.

We were able to make my ma this larger-than-life character who, every time she opened her mouth, a punchline came out. With a great actor like Katherine Lynch we could present a heightened, theatrical image of the person my ma was, someone with a really good sense of humour who looked after loads of people. We could give the character her best qualities and none of her worst. She came out of that show looking like a hero.

It's like stand-up. When you're doing stand-up, you can give the audience a heightened version of who you are for an hour, someone you hope they can relate to. Then for the other twenty-three hours of the day you can go back to being your everyday self.

With a book, though, when you put everything down in black and white, it's so much more open to interpretation. It's a longer, more detailed story and you can't influence what the reader will make of it in the same way you can with a live show. It's more open to the reader's interpretation. So I was afraid that people would only focus on the bad bits and ignore all the good. That worried me because my ma really did incredible things in extraordinary circumstances.

My mother died in November 2022 and they say you can defame the dead but you can't insult them. Neither of these things is my intention in writing this book; I loved my ma probably more than I loved anyone in my life. But I want to tell the story of how I grew up honestly, and since she has died, I'm now free to do that.

It was during the promotion of touring the play back in 2019 that I began to change how I do interviews. I used to think I had to be entertaining. 'This is my job and if I'm not entertaining, I won't get gigs and if I don't get gigs, I can't get fed and if I can't get fed, I can't support myself and I'm screwed.' So, I would think, 'What should I say for this to be a funny interview?'

Then, when I started talking about the events in the play – my experiences as a kid – I could see people's eyes popping out of their heads. That's when I realized that although it all seemed fairly normal to me, it didn't seem remotely normal to them.

So now I just tell people about my life and how I'm feeling, and it works a lot better. Telling stories as they are, or at least the best way I can remember them. No doubt some relatives and family friends will read this book and say, 'That's not how it happened at all.' And I suppose through their eyes, they're right too. But this is how I saw it. This is how it happened for me.

The person whose reaction to this book means most to me is Stacey. She was dying to read the first draft, to see what the madhouse looked like from my point of view, because, even though we both grew up in it, we lived such separate lives. After reading it Stacey texted me to say she always felt so guilty about going to Korea after college and leaving me alone in Ireland, dealing with our ma (even though I lived in a few flats here and there, until I was about twenty-eight I mostly still lived at home).

It blew my mind that Stacey would say that. Growing up I always felt so guilty because I could walk out the door and leave the madness behind. I was older, and more rebellious too. I'd say, 'Fuck off' and walk out, whereas she wouldn't do that, she was more inclined to follow the rules. So for all that time, all our adult lives, we've both been carrying this huge guilt that we let the other one down, that we left the other one stranded there. We were in the same house in the same conditions, but we had two completely different perspectives as to what was going on. It just goes to show that everything in this book is my truth as I saw it. If Stacey wrote a book, it would be a completely different book. Probably a darker book, because I think it was even harder on Stacey than it was on me to grow up in that house.

In recent years all Stacey and I really talked about was how best to keep our ma alive. If I'm honest, I thought we'd drift apart once she died. But since the funeral Stacey's been over in the house a good bit sorting things and we're really beginning to find common ground. We are getting to know each other, maybe for the first time, and making a real fist of growing closer to one another now, which is something I didn't think would happen.

Stacey teases me an unmerciful amount about becoming a father. She's only left me alone with her kids twice. The first time I took them to a garage and told them to buy whatever they wanted – anything to keep them quiet; and the second time two of them nearly ran into the sea fully clothed at an ashes-scattering ceremony on Portmarnock Beach.

Her son Tommy supports Bohemians Football Club, same as me, even though Stacey and her husband are long-time Shelbourne FC fans. For ages he was asking Stacey could he go to a Bohs match with me and she kept saying, 'Next time', 'Next time'. Eventually I rang her up to see what the story was.

'Here, how come Tommy can't come to a match with me?'

''Cause I don't trust you to mind him properly, that's why!'

I don't know what she thinks would happen, that I'd leave him behind in the stands or something, but she does not see me as a responsible child-minding person.

It's strange to both of us that we're now going to have this big thing, parenthood, in common. Neither of us could have seen that coming – me becoming a dad of two at forty-eight. She teases me, but she's delighted her kids will have some cousins from her side of the family, and I'm delighted she's raised three babysitters for me and Kelly.

When she read the first page of this book, she was shocked by my perception of her – that she has it all together and doesn't worry, or doesn't go through her life with the same fear and anxiety I have. She sent me this message to include here: *That is what I might portray outwardly but I just hide it all better, because I also have the anxiety and the panic and the fear of the unknown and the catastrophizing every time my kids go out the door. But I do what I was reared to do, which is pretend that everything is okay and I'm in control, even if the reality is very different.*

The truth is nobody survives a childhood like ours without some damage, but it hasn't stopped Stacey building a life for herself and it isn't going to stop me any longer either.

1.
Alien child

Tara was my first pal, my first friend ever in life. His father was a big Alsatian called Tiger.

The story goes that Tiger would go to the shop in Marino and get the paper for me granda every evening. Now, whether this is true or not I don't know. There's a butcher shop between the house and the newsagents and I can't imagine a dog walking past the butcher shop to go and get the *Evening Press*.

Just like Tiger, Tara looked like a wolf and howled like a wolf – *Woooow Woooooowooooooo*. It was the maddest sound from this dog. And everybody loved Tara. They'd come to the house and ask, 'How's the dog?' before they'd ask about anyone else. We had some great dogs down the years, but none that were ever as universally popular as Tara was.

When I was very little, the few things I remember really caring about were Tara, a toy milk cart and for some reason this outrageous purple paisley carpet we had in the sitting room. I used to lie down on two steps going from the sitting room to the kitchen, and Tara would jump over me. That's the first time I remember laughing – me with my little curls and the dog flying over me, a proper big Alsatian.

There was a lot of yellow going on in our house – the wallpaper in the sitting room was a kind of custard colour with oval shapes that looked like lava lamps on it, horrible but totally fitting of the time. We'd a massive TV, a big Grundig yoke with three colour stripes down the front of it. The weight of a telly back then, if you threw one out a second-storey window it would cause an earthquake.

In the kitchen there was blue wallpaper with practically the same design as the custardy yellow one, and for some reason I can remember piles of those blankets with the ribbed edges on them, in pink and green and blue. Everything was clashing all over the place and screaming 1970s at you.

There's a lot of pictures of me in my nappy putting straws on Tara's head from that time. In those early years when we lived in Marino I wasn't allowed out that much, which was the exact opposite to what happened a few years later when I wasn't allowed in very much. So I played with that dog endlessly, until his hips started to go.

He started struggling standing up and sitting down and all this green stuff started coming out of his mickey that he'd lick off like an ice cream. And, understandably, he was howling a lot, who wouldn't be? And then he was gone.

Because he was my very first friend he has to be the reason I get so attached to dogs. Although, I don't know. You can't be sure of anything, can you? I'm hazarding a guess. Like, if we could ask Tara he might say something different and I'd say he'd remember better than me because my childhood was his entire life.

And it was an interesting life.

We had two Egyptian doctors, two brothers, living on the

ground floor above us, so that dog was living in a multicultural Dublin before most of Dublin was. Then there were my parents, and they were never boring. There was the woman on the first floor who always seemed to be topless in the front garden, and just down the street the pub, PJ Gallagher & Son, that my da was drinking into the ground. But these were in fact the normal years, before the madness started.

Our little patch of turf was situated between Parnell Park and Croke Park; Parnell Park is the Dubs' home ground, even though you wouldn't know it because they never play there, and Croke Park is the High Temple of Gaelic games in Ireland.

I grew up right in between the two of them in Marino, on the corner of the Malahide Road. A nice, typical northside Dublin place, one of those places where all the flags and bunting go up on match days. We were close to the sea and the beaches and right beside the city, so I thought we were in the centre of the universe.

As far as I knew we had everything, and even back then, it felt very mixed; people with different-coloured faces, people with different backgrounds and people you didn't know who they were or where they came from. All of us rubbing up alongside each other. Later, when we moved to Clontarf, everyone was the same, but Marino was my New York City, my cultural melting pot.

And the access to the city, the proximity of it. Any time I heard something on the news, I'd know it had happened or was happening somewhere close to us. That's something I really remember as a kid, looking at the news on TV and thinking, 'Wow, we're *there*.' Ireland might have been in the middle of nowhere, but when it came to Ireland, we were right in the thick of it. I was only five years old, scared in my bed on the 14th of February 1981 when the Stardust fire happened. Sirens wailed up and down the Malahide Road all night, and me ma and da kept saying, 'Something's after happening. Something's after happening.'

We lived in the basement but my ma would always deny the fact that we shared Number 62 with other people. For years, whenever it came up in conversation, I'd say, 'We lived on the basement floor,' and she'd say 'Yeah.' Then I'd say, 'Because there were people living on the other floors,' and she'd say 'No.' 'Well, then,' I'd ask her, 'why the hell did we only live in the basement so?' She'd have no answer for that but I'm telling you now, and I'll stake my life on this, there were people living on those other floors.

One of my earliest memories is going up the stairs with Tara to visit the Egyptian doctors. One of the doctors took me into his study and said, 'I'm going to give you something very important.' He gave me a sword from Egypt, a really sacred thing that he said shouldn't even be in Ireland, it was that sacred. Now, he told me, it was my job to make sure nothing happened to it.

When I broke it, I was shocked – I thought, 'I'm after breaking this thing that probably belonged to Tutankhamun or someone.' I was devastated, until I realized it was a plastic letter opener.

On the top floor lived the woman in the nip. I was too young to understand what sex or attraction was, but I couldn't stop looking at the woman in the nip when she was in the front garden in the same way I can't stop looking at puppies now, you know? There was nothing sexual about it, but it was compelling. She wasn't completely in the nip, she was topless but still, nobody did this in the 80s. Even in Spain I don't think they were doing it.

So, there we were with two Egyptian doctors and a woman in the nip all living in Number 62 alongside us and the dog. At some point the doctors' sister, Zsu Zsu, arrived from Egypt to tell them their father had died, and she ended up living there too.

One thing our family has never been is upwardly mobile, even though my ma loved to think we were. Up until the day she died, if anyone asked her, she would tell them that we had always lived in Clontarf. The second one drop of alcohol hit her lips she'd put on her posh Dublin accent, but she wasn't a Dubliner, not really. Her family were all from Tipperary, a place called Lorrha.

It was probably more a 'lorrha' hardship than a 'lorrha' laughs because there were so many of them: thirteen kids or something. One of her siblings, Little Annie, died before ma was even born; her dress caught on fire and she went up in flames in the front room. And my ma, she was the second youngest of all those brothers and sisters, and I think honestly, having a big family is cruel; she had to watch everyone die before her, including her younger sister Stacey.

The family was very Republican and her father, who was anti-Treaty, was on the run for a huge portion of their lives; up until the 60s he was on the proper, proper run. When my grandfather decided to play a bit less hide-and-seek and wind down his active service to Mother Ireland, they moved to Wicklow. You'd have to feel for the man, because he lived through a British-occupied Ireland into an Irish-occupied Ireland, but he still found himself being the enemy. When the family finally made their way to Dublin, he'd use his brother's house in the city to sneak out on his covert operations.

He used his brother's house because his brother was gay

and so men coming and going from the house at all hours didn't raise any suspicions with the guards. According to my mother, the only people out late at night back in the 60s were the gay men and the gunmen.

But my grandfather wasn't the only one sneaking around on covert missions. His daughter, Helen Gallagher *née* Kirwan, could be a bit of a shady character herself.

Just after her funeral me and Stacey were going through this and that and we found her passport. We were like, 'That doesn't look like Ma in the picture, it's more like Auntie Ann.' We asked one of our cousins who said, 'Oh, did you not know? Your ma forged that passport so she could pretend she was our ma and start nursing in Liverpool at fourteen instead of sixteen.'

So she never qualified as a nurse under her own name, she qualified under her sister's name, and we only found out literally the week after she died when we found her fake passport.

Growing up she used to tell us these mad stories about her younger days. She famously went out with Seamus Costello, who ended up being the founding member of the IRSP* and their buddies, the INLA.† The IRSP are the Sinn Féin of the INLA, its political wing. The last time she met him, she had me in her arms, and soon after he was shot on North Circular Road and killed. So she knew all kinds of everybody in the world, she really did.

Later when I joined Sinn Féin and she was dropping me into the meetings, it used to break her heart. At this point she just thought it wasn't worthwhile and it turns out she was right, it wasn't worthwhile, it was a waste of time.

* Irish Republican Socialist Party.
† Irish National Liberation Army.

My father, Sean Gallagher, grew up in Dublin but his family was the complete opposite, much smaller, only him and his sister Eileen. Eileen ended up living in Cork where I went on my holidays, down to Auntie Eileen's. She was one of those aunties that, in fairness to her, you do have to give her credit because she was always on her way up to see you, but she would never turn up.

'I'm up there next week. Next week. I will be in Dublin next week, and I'll drop in to you.'

You'd know you wouldn't have to put that date in the diary. Then, if she ever did drop in, it'd be completely unexpected, no warning shot. Which is a weird way to behave, isn't it? My personal philosophy on visitors: fire a flare or fuck off.

My father's mother, Lily, she was a Cocoman from Offaly before she got married and became a Gallagher. Cocoman is such an unusual kind of name that doesn't really fit with Ireland. It always makes me think of Kid Creole, who used to sing with a band called The Coconuts. We called Lily 'Ma'am' (like the royal 'Ma'am') and my mam would be 'Ma'. The two of them did not get on, not even a bit, which suited me down to the ground.

Whenever I was in trouble bars of chocolate came flying out of Granny's bag. Which was great. I was her favourite, big time. There was no doubt about it. When the cousins were around, no matter what treats were being doled out, she'd always have a little extra for me. I was delighted. I loved Granny's visits. Granny's visits were the business.

By the time I got curious about how my parents met, my da was dead and me ma was at the age where she couldn't answer a question without starting at the end. By the time she'd get to the beginning I didn't care any more. That's the problem with getting older: you hit an age where you've stories to tell, knowledge and information to impart, but for some reason your delivery has gone to hell.

All I do know is that they were married by Father Michael Cleary and The Wolfe Tones played at the reception and when they tried to start a family they couldn't. Hazarding a guess, I'd say it was dangerous. It was the 70s, right? So there was a lot of pubic hair, a lot of friction fires, people being removed from each other in hospitals. And they were married a fair while before they adopted me, so it's possible they got to the stage where they wanted children but looked at each other and thought, 'You know, I haven't seen you in the nip since 1962. Let's go to the orphanage.'

It was just easier to adopt back then. They didn't grill you the way they do now. I think there were maybe about three questions: *Have you ever been in jail for more than ten years?* No. *Are you gay?* Don't be ridiculous, there's no gay people in Ireland. *Do you go to Mass?* Yeah. *Okay, so, a boy or a girl?*

Gallagher family legend goes that I was delivered to my father's pub. There was no one in the house so they brought me up to the pub. I've always had this image of some fella pulling up with a load of babies and going:

'Here, Sean, was it a boy or a child you were getting?' and my da saying, 'A boy.'

'Right you are, here's your kid.'

Throwing me at my da, who says to him, 'D'you wanna stop for a pint?' and him saying, 'No I can't, I've five more kids to deliver sitting in the car. Anyway, if I don't get home before six o'clock, I'll be getting all that from the missus.'

It can't be true but it's a good story.

There's an awful lot of fantasy involved in being an adopted kid. There's no doubt about that. Fantasy is your friend. As a kid I spent a lot of time thinking, 'Okay, if I didn't come from these people, who or what did I come from?' It's a game you play in your head all the time. Because you're trying to fit in all the time, and when things aren't going your way, or things aren't going to plan, there's an opt-out in your head that goes, 'Well, one day my alien parents will come back from whatever planet they're on and show me how to use my superpowers.'

I used to think like that all the time, right into my teens, just as a fantasy, but especially when I was a kid. Aliens were a big thing for me.

'There's definitely aliens out there, and they left me here for safekeeping. Maybe the ship was wrecked or maybe they died in a crater and I've got some great alien cousin that looks exactly like me and will turn up some day and collect me.'

As if aliens look like boggers who get really bad neck sunburn in July.

But I would think like that all the time. Convinced I had superpowers and just didn't know how to use them yet.

Running and sprinting and taking those bigger strides, and thinking, 'I've just about figured this out. I'm just about to take off here.'

Wondering, in the days before email and the Nigerian Prince, if there was a chest of millions out there that I would inherit some day. Because you really do think that your parents could be anyone. Even mad killers who had to hide me somewhere so I wouldn't have to go on the run with them.

There was one outcome I wanted more than anything else if I ever did find them, if they ever did come looking. More than aliens, more than superheroes, I wanted them to be Americans. If you had given me the choice between aliens, superheroes or Americans I'd have picked Americans all day long. That's what I wanted the most. To go and live in Americaland. In the telly, where the superstars were. Americans were the coolest. In fact, Americans practically *were* superheroes.

Of course, little did I know, at the time, Irish kids were being sold to Americans by the Catholic Church. Because in Ireland, adoption was big business back in those days. And there were that many spare kids you couldn't give them away.

One time I was in the car with me da, messing around, being a little tosser, shouting, 'Pass them out! Pass them out!' My da stopped on the Malahide Road beside the Travellers' encampment and said to a man there, 'Here listen, are you looking for a young fella, 'cause I've had enough of this one.'

The man was clued in and went, 'Ah, he looks a bit weak, I've a five-year-old here who can change the engine out of a van, I don't know what I'd do with that one.'

Now I was *losing* it in the back seat. After all, I was given away once, so the idea of being given away a second time scared the hell out of me. And then the man says, 'Ah no, look, I've enough mouths to feed,' and my da goes, 'All right, I'll give him one more chance.'

There was no cloak and dagger stuff in our house around adoption, so I never had to find out, something I'm very grateful for. I know a fella whose folks only told him when he was eighteen and it was too much for him. To me it was normal to the point of being boring.

The first time I realized being adopted was unusual was in primary school. I was talking to a lad and suddenly the penny dropped, he was with the parents who gave birth to him. This was shocking to me and I thought, *Jaysus, this guy, nobody wants him, poor fella has to stay with his first family*.

When you get adopted there's this six-month probation period during which your birth mother can pick up the phone and say, 'I want my child back,' and you have to give them back, that's just the rule.

When I found out about that I said to my mother, 'What would you have done, like if you got that call, what would you have done?'

And she said, 'Oh, I'd have given you back in a heartbeat, yeah. Straight away. Stuck a tenner in your nappy, put you in a taxi, gone.'

I was absolutely raging with her. 'Why? Like what in the name of God would you have done that for?'

And she told me the story. The last time she was ever in the adoption agency they sat her down and said, 'We've found a child for you, we've found a boy.' She was over the moon, the happiest she had probably ever been in her life up to then. She couldn't wait to tell my father. But just before she left, she saw a woman who was in a bad way crying. It sort of stuck with her that maybe the woman was the mother of the child she was about to get. And the thought never left her.

2.
Meet the parents

One day, out of the blue, I had a sister. I must have been very busy that day playing with the dog or putting a hole in the carpet because I don't remember her arrival. There was no transition, no one was pregnant or anything. Just one day when I was nearly three I walked into the front room and there was a cot in the corner of the room just under the window. And I looked into the cot and there was a baby in it.

'Who's that?' And me da was like, 'That's your sister.'

'Is it?'

'Yeah, that's your sister.'

'Is she gonna live here?'

'Yeah, your sister's gonna live here.'

Relatives arrived to see the new baby and I was walking around holding my sister in my arms like a prize turkey saying, 'Have you met me new sister? She's brand new!'

No one told kids anything back then and me da, he never said anything about anything. It was a constant battle for the man's attention. I don't remember him saying anything to me about being adopted other than: 'You're our son, and that's the end of it.' And when we fell out: 'You're not my son.'

Grand, if that's the way you want it.

So there wasn't a huge amount of dialogue there. There was never a huge amount of dialogue.

For instance, it was a terrible shock when I found out my name stood for something. Before that I thought it was just the letters P and J stuck together, and it was a teacher who told me they weren't letters but initials. We had a big fight about it because I just thought PJ was a name like Brian or Andrew or Keith. When I went home my ma had to explain to me that it stood for Patrick Joseph. Patrick because he was the patron saint of Ireland and we were Irish first and foremost, and Joseph because when Holy God got Mary pregnant Joseph came over to Holy God and said, 'Look, I know you've a lot on your plate, you go off and do your God things and I'll look after the baby God.' By default, that then made Joseph the first adoptive father in history.

I went into my da and said, 'Da, I just found out how I got my name,' and told him the story and he said, 'That's a load of rubbish, you're named after my da.'

That's just the way the man was, he didn't mince his words. The reason I found out there was no Santa was because he took me down to the bike shop and said, 'Which one of these do you want Santa to get you?'

All right, I thought, *so that's how that works.*

I'm the image of my da, so no one ever believed I was adopted. We even have the same voice. I don't know how he did it, did he come into my room when I was asleep and squish me face up and sort of like set it with a load of plastic bands till it looked like his?

My father, I think, was a fellow who tried to tick the boxes of what he thought he was supposed to do. He said he wanted to be a pilot, but he wasn't allowed. I suppose saying he wanted to be a pilot when he was young would be like me, now, in my forties, saying, 'I want to be an Olympic gymnast.' It was a ludicrous aspiration back then. Not going to happen.

Instead, he was taken out of school at fourteen and made to work in the family pub and I think he just spent his life trying to impress people after that. Trying to do the right thing. Telling everybody what they wanted to hear.

'Do you agree with this?'

'Yes.'

He agreed with everything. No matter what people said, he would agree with it.

I've got a picture of me and him on the beach from when I was a kid. I'm on the beach in my nip because that used to be grand. I've nothing on but a pair of armbands and me da, he's standing beside me with a comb-over and a cigarette, dressed in a full suit.

I look at that picture now and I think, 'What happened to that man?' He must have just thought that was the way you deal with life: you got married, had kids, wore a suit to the beach and hoped for the best.

It must be remarkable to think you're doing everything you're supposed to do, and then to still feel very unfulfilled afterwards. And he was very unfulfilled. I know he was. I mean, the man got drunk every day. And it wasn't a party.

I think he was embarrassed about things and wanted people to think he was doing well. Needed people to think he was a good guy. Needed kudos.

I meet people all the time who tell me, 'Your da was such

a great guy.' And I'm like, 'Was he? I wish I knew because I couldn't get a word out of him.'

There was always this question about whether he spoke Irish or not. I'd ask him, 'Do you speak Irish?'

'Yeah.'

'Do you read it?'

'No.'

Whatever I asked him, there'd be no conversation, no chat. He seemed to chat to everyone outside the house and no one in the house.

And yet I meet people all the time that are like, 'You're just like him.' I'm like, 'Me? I never shut my bloody mouth!' They're like, 'Yeah. Just like him.' The person they knew and the person I knew are two totally different people, and I can't work it out.

The best way I can describe him is that he was like a ghost. I always felt I was more haunted by my old man than lived with him.

Effectively it was me ma that looked after us, for better or for worse. She was very defensive of us and she worried about us, worried too much. When I started walking to school on my own, she used to follow me and jump into gardens to watch me. One half of her watching to see if I was going to do what I was told and the other half to see would I go off with the first man that had a puppy and a bag of sweets.

She had a real caring and forgiving nature that was, I suppose, her best feature. No matter what I did, or my old man did, or she did for that matter, she would find a way of forgiving us all. So, I mean, you could rob a post office – not that anyone ever did that I'm aware of – you could rob a post office and come into the house and say, 'I robbed a post office, there's like a hundred grand upstairs.'

All she'd say would be, 'Make it disappear,' and the next day, you'd wake up, everything forgotten.

Every morning in our house was like that, like nothing had happened the day before. She and me da would get locked some nights and tear the house asunder and you'd hear 'em getting sick or roaring at each other and saying things that would be normal relationship enders.

Then everyone would wake up and it was like, 'How are ya, love, nice to see you this morning.' It was bananas, really weird. It was Groundhog Day every day. The world would start out fine every morning and then end in an absolute tornado.

But you could rely on her not to sweat the big stuff – like robbing post offices or dropping out of school at sixteen. Things that might send most other people's parents around the bend she took in her stride.

Ma liked to say she never hit any of us, but she tried very hard to batter me with a tennis racket in the garden once. Me and my friend Peter had built a cart and wanted to paint it but I couldn't open the can, so I just thought I'd smash it with a hammer. The paint went everywhere, all over my da's shed, and I knew I was going to be in trouble, so I said to Peter, 'Here's what we'll do. Instead of trying to clean it up, 'cause that won't work, we'll piss the paint out the door.'

Somehow, I thought that by the power of our piss we could piss the paint out the door. Then, if it's in the garden and not inside, anyone could have spilled it! But the force of piss didn't work, so I went into the house and got one of my ma's rugs and put it on top of the piss-paint cocktail. When she came into the shed and lifted the rug she went mental, grabbed a tennis racket and just started swinging. She hit the floor, she hit the walls, she hit Peter a few times, but she somehow missed me. Till the day she died she'd say, 'I'll give myself credit for one thing. When you were growing up I never hit yiz, not one time.' And it's true. But only because she missed.

Well, whatever, these things happen and I don't think it had anything to do with me having a weird childhood or there being a load of drink in the house. I just think, unfortunately, people want to hit people when they get angry sometimes.

Every time she gave out to us, she felt guilty over it. You could always see the guilt on the horizon, even if we deserved it. She'd scream at you, throw you into your room, and then come up and give you a bar of chocolate and stay for a chat.

The one time she did lock me in my room, she hadn't wanted to do it. I must have been spectacularly bad that day, because my granny, who usually doted on me, said to her, 'You need to lock that child up the way he's carrying on, the way he's speaking to me. If your husband spoke to me that way when he was a boy, I'd have put his head through the wall.'

Because she was always afraid of being judged by my granny, she brought me upstairs to my room, closed the door and told me she'd locked it. Well, of course, I immediately set my escape into action, looked out the window of the house and realized that if I could hang off the window, I could drop on to the garage roof. And I did. Then I ran to the kitchen window, gave me granny the finger and climbed up the willow tree down the back of the garden.

And me ma, she ran out screaming at me to come down from the tree, which I didn't want to do because I was afraid of getting battered. And she was like, 'I didn't even lock the bloody door!' So, even at those times she still couldn't find it within herself to really punish us.

She punished people around us a lot more than she ever punished us. One teacher wrongly accused me of robbing a bike and, Jesus, did he live to regret it.

I suppose I did have a bad reputation. I was terrible in school in every single way. And then when you're told often enough you're useless and bad, you start trying to live up to it. (Years later, when I came home from school at the beginning of fourth year and said I wanted to leave she was like, 'Oh, thank God.' She had a pain in her ass going into the school. Every time she was up there she would ask if there were any other PJ Gallaghers because she found it really difficult to believe one person could be in that much trouble.)

Anyway, I hadn't robbed anyone's bike and my ma went in with a few jars on her and tore strips off the teacher in front of the class. I kind of wish I had been there for that, because I've only ever heard the stories about what it was like. I really wish I had gotten to see that sort of legendary dressing-down, because most of the time she embarrassed me with this kind of carry-on. But it sounded epic.

For all the boozing, my ma wasn't far off ninety when she died. At one point I thought, *D'you know what, I'll probably die before her and probably in a drink-related accident!* I could just hear her saying, 'Poor fella, he wasn't doing it right, that's the problem. He wasn't practised enough. He only drank on the weekends.'

3.
PJ Gallagher & Son

Our pub was 'PJ Gallagher & Son', and it was a proper 80s pub with carpet on the floors. Whose idea was that? The carpet had black tar-like tufts on it that still to this day I don't know was it chewing gum or just muck off shoes that landed there and decided to stay forever. There were these natty red leather chairs with steel legs on them, the sort of thing you'd never see in a pub now, and red leather couches. The couches were the type that went around corners and were over-inflated at the front. On the walls there were a lot of paintings of the pub, Dublin football jerseys, replica trophies and jerseys of the football team sponsored by the pub in the local league.

One of my earliest memories is of the time the pub was chosen to display the Sam Maguire Cup. It was a big deal, there were a lot of players and I was just a little kid, dressed in all the Dublin gear. But the adults, for some reason they thought a great way to celebrate would be to fill the Sam Maguire Cup up with alcohol and shove me in it, just throw me in, like an olive in a cocktail glass.

I was terrified, like genuinely afraid for my life. Someone took a photograph of the ordeal, and my folks thought it would be fitting to frame that photograph and hang it on the wall. A framed picture on the pub wall of me being jeered at by adults, crying and just generally bringing the tone down. It's a miracle I'm still a fan of the Dublin team.

The pub was always open all hours because me da, he'd hate to deprive someone of a drink or a bit of company.

'What can I bleedin' do? I'll have to give him a drink, the man wants a drink, you know what I mean?'

Essentially me aul man was a dealer and his customers were addicts. And because it was the 70s and 80s it was totally okay for kids to rock around the pub all day long. There were no child-minders, you didn't get dropped off somewhere, and there were no playdates. So I'd sit around with addicts at six and seven like a little old man.

'All right, Jimmy.'

'Ah, how are ya, PJ? Did you get the new toy?'

'I did, Jimmy. Thanks for asking. How are you getting on yourself?'

'Grand, PJ, grand. Can't complain.'

Hanging out in the pub all day being fed doorstop cheese sandwiches, packets of crisps and loads of fizzy drinks. Hanging out and having these proper conversations with professional alcoholics, drinking seven Lucozades and then getting in trouble because I couldn't sit down. 'That child never stops moving, Jesus Christ, where does he get his energy from?'

From the seven bottles of Lucozade and the fucking non-stop crisps and sandwiches, that's where.

In pubs back then you could go in and get a rotisserie chicken. Do you remember? You can't do that any more, sit down and eat a full chicken with a pint. My ma always told me, 'Your father brought the rotisserie chicken to the pubs of Ireland.' This is at an age when I thought everything was very impressive. I spent a lot of time hanging out in the pub listening to my old pair brag about rotisserie chickens. It is definitely not a true story.

Booze was always a presence and a problem in our lives, not that I knew drink was the problem, I just assumed adults got a bit nasty after dark. I'd be playing with my toys in the pub or whatever and they'd interrupt me and say, 'Go up there and get us a brandy and ginger ale and a vodka and tonic, will ya.' I wasn't pouring the drinks, but I was getting the order in the same way your dad might ask you to change the channel on the TV.

It was all spirits back then. I remember that. There was a shift, later in their lives, when they decided to try and take it a bit handy and go from the whiskey to the wine and the vodka to the Guinness. But in those early days my father was a vodka maniac.

Sometimes my aul fella would park the car outside some pub after a match and say he'd only be a minute and you'd know you were going to be sitting in the car on your own for four or five hours.

One time I was walking home to the house as a teenager and I saw my old man walking towards me, so I knew immediately there was a problem. My da never walked. However short the distance, he'd sooner drive the car at ten mile an hour than actually walk it. I went straight up to him: 'What's the problem?'

'The car's been robbed. I was in the pub and now . . . and now it's gone.'

'How long were you in the pub for?'

'Twenty minutes.'

'Yeah, right. Give us the keys to the car, I'll go look for the car. Give me the keys.'

'It doesn't matter about the keys to the car now, does it? Because there is no car.'

When I went down to the pub the car was literally in arm's reach of the pub door. I was raging at the man for being so stupid. Then, pulling into the driveway I nearly killed him. Just in time, I saw two legs sticking out of one of my ma's rose bushes. He was lying there face down, it was as if he was standing to attention, but on his nose. Face down in the rose bushes. I went up to him and said, 'What are you doing?'

'I'm looking for something.'

'What do you mean you're looking for something, what are you looking for?'

'The keys to the car.'

Alcohol was everything. Birthdays were just an excuse for everyone to get even more plastered; uncles, most of the aunties, everyone coming around plastered at a seven-year-old's birthday or communion or confirmation. Anything like that was an excuse for an absolute all-day session. Not that the excuse was needed. I used to dread people coming to the gaff because you knew this is it now. This is it. Now it starts and it doesn't end.

That's how they socialized, they just got smashed.

One Christmas, I was four or five, and we were all in the front room above the pub. The adults were doing that thing Irish adults do instead of dancing, they were holding hands and going round in circles singing 'Brown Girl in the Ring'.

Now for some reason I was the brown girl in the ring with these mad drunk adults dancing in circles around me.

Terrifying. Then from the corner of my eye, I saw it . . . you know in those old films your man has a rifle and he's about to shoot an antelope then something makes him look over his shoulder and there's an elephant running at him and he freezes? Well, in this scene I'm the fella with the rifle and my Uncle Gerry is the charging elephant. He was running at me hard. But it turned out he wasn't running. He was trying to stay on his feet, and he had his hand on his chest and making this terrible noise –

Huuuuuh . . .

Huuuuuuuuuuuh . . .

He took about three steps and collapsed right on top of me. Now he was a small man, but I was a little child and I hit the deck, the full weight of a grown man lying across my face and chest. I tried to scream GET OFF! but I couldn't because the weight was so hard.

It took only about three seconds for someone to pull me out but it felt like three hours. The next day everyone was at the table saying what a terrible thing it was about Gerry's heart attack. 'Terrible thing, terrible thing.' Terrible thing my hole. *I* nearly died of Uncle Gerry's heart attack after him pinning me to the ground like Hulk Hogan. There were nearly two of us that went with the same heart.

Gerry survived for years after it, he worked as a barman in Eamon Doran's until his fourth heart attack finally killed him. But I wasn't around for those other three.

Bobby Rice was another uncle of mine and was one of the gayest men I've ever met, although he never came out of the closet. This is a man who in his nineties didn't need a cane because he just floated along the ground. That's how camp he was. His son Johnny, who was a lovely kid, was gay as well; an insanely posh, camp kid (and adopted like me, something I only found out recently). Any time he came to our house, if my ma would get on his nerves, he'd go, 'That's it, I'm getting a taxi.' And he'd walk out of the house and get a taxi. In the 80s! He always had this fifty-pound note, he'd be waving it in the air singing, 'I'm getting a taxi.' Sadly, Johnny died in his sleep nearly fifteen years ago now.

Uncle Bobby owned Rice's Pub on Stephen's Green and I was in that bar so much as a kid, I loved it. It wasn't until I was an adult that I realized it was one of the first gay bars in the country, or 'gay-friendly' bars as they used to say. We'd go into town during the day, have a wander round the old Dandelion Market and then into Rice's, everyone leaving it drunk later that night. One night coming home from there we had a crash; the back seat of the car came out and crushed me under its weight. When I eventually got out from under it, I remember seeing this man walking around. I thought he was shot but he must have just hit his head off something, there was blood crawling down his face like lightning bolts.

Whenever I'd ask my ma, 'Do you remember that car crash?' she'd say back to me, 'We were never in a car crash. Never. We were never, ever in a car crash.'

Now, I also remember her nearly ramming a bus off the Malahide Road but apparently that didn't happen either. It was like that in our house, no one ever confirmed anything because, I suppose, nothing ever happened, and I was making it all up?

In a pub, any pub, if you're in it enough, you'll see chaos. And if you're a kid in a pub you see adult drama long before you know what adult drama even is. Then there's the people trying to share their drinks with you, aul fellas asking, 'D'you want some of this?'

They'd no idea how to talk to kids other than, 'D'you want some of this?'

But I don't hate pubs, I love pubs, I'm just terrified of the control alcohol has, what it can do to people, but pubs I love in the same way I love rollercoasters and motorbikes. Everybody that goes to a pub is playing with fire, they're just used to it.

You know how in the 1950s cars had those seatbelts that only went across your lap and if you had an accident they could literally sever your body in half? That's the way I see pubs: they're 1950s cars with lap belts and they're really dangerous. They can ruin your life in a heartbeat but there's quite a lot of enjoyment to them at the same time.

Going to the pub is a strange activity because you walk in and you see the tragedy. In every pub you can see the tragedy, but you don't care, you just carry on. There's no other activity in life you can say that about.

If you walked towards a rollercoaster, and there were people with severed limbs lying around the bottom screaming because they got seriously hurt or someone had fallen off and died, you wouldn't get on the rollercoaster.

But you'll go into a pub with proper addicts and alcoholics sitting around, very obvious, and you'll go, 'Rack us up a pint there.'

It's a bit mad. We throw caution to the wind when we walk into the pub. I don't know why we do it? It's more than just cultural but probably there is a bit of 'You won't tell me what to do' about it.

And, the fact of the matter is, there's not very many things you can do that'll give you a buzz and a bit of a release that easily.

You know when people say, 'When was the first time you had a pint with your old man?' Well, we had the same pint and we were literally sharing it and I don't know what age I was, but

I was young. I don't even know if I'd started school. I was sitting at the bar and I had this black robot toy with me. You stuck little red missiles into him, pressed a button on his head, and they would not fly off, they would fall off. It was crap. The telly was on, the horse racing, and he gave me some of his pint to show me how terrible it was so I would never have a pint again. Well, well, well. What a failed experiment that was!

4.

Holy Faith, Evel Knievel and Americaland

People who've been adopted can often remember their christening day, because even though someone would have 'officially' christened you at the hospital your new family usually like to have their own day out, and by that stage you'd be a bit older than a baby. My folks took this to the extreme, of course, and waited until Stacey arrived to christen us together, a two-for-the-price-of-one deal. So I walked into my own christening when I was about three and a half years old, into the church my folks got married in and my sister would too, years later.

No one would tell me what was going on that day, so there I was up on the altar holding a candle and complaining that it's not even Sunday, it's Saturday and what were we doing at Mass? Asking me da over and over again what was going on and him just saying, 'Ah, you know, yourself.' But I didn't know, did I? I was only three!

I was very easily bribed, however.

'We're going to McDonald's after.'

Grand.

They'd dressed me in these little shorts that would look good on someone in a nightclub today – a little sort of army faux canvas jacket with deep pockets and little shoulder tassels. It was an amazing outfit and my hair looked like a banger went off on my head. I looked like a little girl, a great little girl. Which didn't bother me too much and just as well; being dressed up as a girl was something I was going to have to get used to.

My folks had left it so long to register me for primary school that by the time they did, the only one I could get into was Holy Faith Girls' School. At Holy Faith me and four other boys were the only boys in the whole school. They put us in big yellow smocks to keep our pants and T-shirts clean, so I was wearing a dress I suppose. But I didn't have any gender knowledge or awareness at the time, so I didn't care, I was just a young lad looking like everyone else.

There's only one picture of me at Holy Faith and for some reason they put me in the middle with all the girls around me. We're in our Communion outfits, me in a tux and the girls in their white dresses. There are other lads in the photo but they're all at the sides, so when you crop them out I look like a cult leader surrounded by his thirty wives.

There's nothing to do in Junior Infants except draw with crayons and look out the window. I remember doing some sort of art thing that very first day and being completely bored out of my mind, and I stayed that way until I left school at sixteen. School was just a horrendous, boring, never-ending penance for me.

Even as a five-year-old I remember dragging my ass out of bed and pulling my jeans up over my George Best underwear, getting in the back of the car, or worse still, having to walk up the road to school. Then sitting down at a desk in a classroom and just waiting for this unbelievable torture of a day in a fancy school in Clontarf to end.

The principal was a nun and she had all the characteristics to be a villain in a book like *Matilda*. She didn't like children very much, never mind boys; she was there to educate the girls, not the ridiculous boys wearing smocks and doing art projects. Especially not boys like me, with no interest in the place.

Some people will shout at you no matter what you do, and I was in trouble with her all the time, but I never remember doing anything much except for one incident. We were copying letters and I had never cared less about anything in my life. So, I half-arsed it. Even in Junior Infants I was half-arsing stuff and I've made a whole career out of half-arsing everything since. (On our radio show at Nova, my co-host Jim does all the work. It's a running joke that my sole purpose on that show is to turn up and lighten the mood. All I want to do is get in, have fun and go home. The other day my friend Damien told me I only work from the neck up and it's true. I'm as lazy as a shot dog.)

She picked up my bit of paper and gave me my first assessment. According to her, my work was ridiculously lazy and a huge insult to all the girls in the class, some of whom were still working hard on their letters. It was annoying but I didn't care that much. What I learnt that day is that it's much easier to be in trouble than to make an effort.

Not one time at school did I ever do homework; it's so much easier to just go in and get in trouble for ten minutes than it is to sit at home for an hour doing something you've no interest in. And trust me, if you persist, they will give up on you. And it's worth it, you know? Like it's really worth it.

So, if you're a kid reading this, take my advice. Homework

is pointless and you're going to get to a stage in your life where it'll just give you the bad habit of taking your work home with you. Persist with idleness until people give up on you! That's the best advice I can share with anybody.

The other big memory I have from being in Holy Faith Girls' School is throwing my pencil case at Simon B. It was shaped like a guitar and when you put pencils in they looked like the strings of the guitar. We were doing some exercise and Simon was making faces at me, insinuating I was stupid. The more he did it the more I could feel the anger rising in me.

Like a kid would, I asked him to stop a few times: 'Please don't you be making faces at me.' I'm speculating, but I think somebody teasing me for being stupid when I was only at single-digit age hit me where it hurt, because from the beginning I felt very inadequate at school, very out of place.

When he did it again, I lost my mind and threw the Spanish guitar pencil case at him. The zip cut his face and when you're that little and you see blood it's very dramatic. I thought I'd killed him. The trouble I got into over it. The teachers were giving out saying, 'We'll call your parents,' but I was much more afraid of Simon being hurt than I was of being in trouble at home or at school.

The first girl I ever fell for was a girl in my class called Aran. I think it was the last year I was there, which was Communion year, so I was about seven or eight. My Jesus. I didn't realize that I fancied her, I just knew I had to be beside her. Finally, there was a reason that school wasn't a complete misery.

Around the same time *The A-Team* was on telly and it was all the lads were talking about. All of a sudden, school wasn't the worst place in the whole world to be, you know? I talked to the other boys about *The A-Team*, and then I sat down and looked at Aran for the day.

There was another girl in the class whose name I can't remember, but one day one of the teachers asked me to do something and this girl said, 'If you can stop looking at Aran for five minutes.'

Oh my God, the shame. That was the first time I ever felt real shame. SHAME SHAME. I genuinely thought my heart was gonna stop. Everybody laughed and, my God, it was awful.

Sometimes Aran and I would sit holding hands, just looking at each other. We had no idea what was going on. It was just that feeling of wanting to be around someone, discovering that you like people who aren't like you. But the minute that girl teased me the bubble burst.

Up until seven, eight, I hadn't been around boys very much and so the big fear at the time was going to a school with boys in it, which we had to do after Communion. The boys in our school, we didn't really hang out with each other. We hung out with the girls and we all had our own groups of friends. Like, we didn't just hang out with each other because we were little lads with flutes.

Oh, the panic. I can still feel it. Knowing I was going to leave this world and spend all day every day with boys. I remember begging and begging my parents, 'Please don't send me to a boys' school, please don't send me to a boys' school!'

'But there is no other girls' school that's gonna take you!'

So I moved to Belgrove in Clontarf for the rest of primary, even though I was terrified of being around other lads. It worked out fine. But I still absolutely despised being in a school environment.

*

Growing up in the 80s there were all these urban legends going around about how much money could be made as an altar boy. Rumours about a lad who did a funeral and got fifty quid, another lad who did a wedding and got thirty quid and you were like, *Oh man, that is a brilliant gig!* The opportunity to make a few quid is the only reason anyone does it, no matter what they tell you. When I started the gig, I realized I'd been in Mass my whole life and I still had no idea what was going on, bar the usual:

'He broke bread, gave it to the disciples and said –'

All that sort of stuff.

'The Mass has ended, go in peace to love and serve the Lord.'

That one everyone knew because the response was 'Thank Christ for that!'

Christenings were brilliant, not as wordy as weddings and funerals, so you didn't have to do much. The priest went solo at christenings.

But the rest of the time you were the backing singer. You had to remember where to come in. That was the hard part of being an altar boy, it's so easy to zone out, there's not a lot more boring than Mass. Every week I forgot everything: when to ring the bell, when to go backstage and get all the props, the water and Jesus Juice. I never got it right. Not even once. There I'd be, listening to a priest mumbling whatever it is they mumble, and trying to remember to ring the bell when he lifted up the big Jesus crisp – not like the little ones he'd give out to the people at communion, but the Daddy Jesus crisp – and still almost every single time I'd forget to ring the bell. The priest would look over all upset so then I'd have to ring it. Late.

But I always persevered, thinking I'd get a few quid out of

it, even putting up with them dressing me like a little priest, wearing the surplice and satin.

Nothing makes an altar boy happier than a death in the local community. You got loads of money for funerals and weddings but especially funerals. Catch someone distracted by grief and they're very likely to give you a few quid. At weddings there's a bit more of a budget, they've a lot of things to pay for and they're thinking 'I'm already paying seventeen quid to feed these animals beef or salmon.' You'd make a few bob but not loads. At funerals, though, they'd be crying and emptying their pockets into your hands. You were young, so a spate of aul ones and aul fellas disappearing off the face of the earth was nothing; as far as you were concerned they'd already been alive for 232 years or something.

During Fr Houlihan's tenure, whatever money you made, you kept. Fr Houlihan was sound. He drove what looked like a sports car and was a proper rock star in the area. Then Fr Larkin took over, the big old, dirty, holy-box that he was. Larkin decided he was keeping all the money and at the end of the year it would go towards a trip for us all. We were looking forward to it, thinking we'd be going to Galway at the very least. But he took us to Bray. This was pre-DART. It didn't come until 1984. So we got on to a poxy little coach, went out to Bray, walked up to the top of Bray Head, came down, got a 50 pence piece each, and then went on the bumpers.

I was raging. I was like, 'We have been ripped off, absolutely ripped off!' A year's work for 50 pence! I worked all them weddings and funerals and christenings and my only reward was going on a bus to Bray to walk up a hill? The hill is free, you pricks! No one fell for that, nobody fell for it.

Like honestly, I'm still upset about it. Even when I was in that church with me ma and me da at their funerals and the coffins were coming up the aisle to go back into the hearse, I was thinking, *These scabby chancers owe me money.*

My da taught me how to cycle, and just that first experience when you go on a bike with no stabilizers, you know that feeling when he's holding the back of the seat and he's like, 'Go, go, go, go, go' and then you realize that he's not there any more and you panic and fall off. You scare the life right out of yourself but you go, *Jesus, I'm gonna do that again.*

The stabilizers weren't long off the bike when my Uncle Matt put some 50 pences on the grass and told me to cycle by and see if I could pick them up. Uncle Matt, my mother's brother, was an interesting character, a proper eccentric. He became a priest late in life and travelled the world. He was like Uncle 'Traveling' Matt from *Fraggle Rock*, except human and a priest. Whenever you met him, he bellowed 'Hel-loooooooooooo' at you. *Hellooooooooooooooooo?* He was LOUD. A wild man with the maddest, poshest accent, huge boots on his feet and big bushes of hair sticking out the side of an otherwise bald head.

Before he became a priest he had owned the Dalkey Island Hotel, but he drank it into the sea, crashed a car and found God. This was a fella who claimed to have put the goats out on Dalkey Island, him and my ma; I can only imagine it, the two of them drunk with a boatful of goats. Although, the more I think about that story the bigger the smell of crap that comes off it.

He put the 50 pence pieces on the ground and at the time I didn't really understand much about gravity and how it works, so when I tried to pick them up, I came off the bike and brained myself, hurt myself proper. But there was something about it; like, *IMAGINE you could pick them up!*

I don't know if the 50 pence stunts with Uncle Matt came before or after I watched re-runs of Evel Knievel on the telly, but from the first moment I saw him flying through the air on his motorbike I was hooked. And even though he turned out to be a bit of a bollox, Evel Knievel is the one idol I've had in my life. I don't know what it was or why he had such an effect on me but it must be connected to that feeling I had, the very first time I was on a bike ever. Something just happened. It felt like this is where I'm supposed to be. A great feeling of 'I'm doing something that I really enjoy.' Even as a little kid with stabilizers I felt that way.

As long as I live I'll never forget watching re-runs of Evel Knievel's 1975 Wembley jump on TV. That interview when he's standing there saying this is the last jump he'll ever do.

'I am done. I quit, it is over.'

There was a story at the time about how he flew into London and decided driving on the left-hand side of the road was stupid. So he just drove on the right in England because 'Americans invented driving and I'm gonna drive like an American.' He was as ignorant, you know? Didn't care that he was in another country with completely different rules. Had no respect for them. I'd say he would have made a terrible dinner guest.

The thing about him was he knew he wasn't going to make most of these jumps, all his big, big jumps. He never made any of them. He didn't make Caesar's Palace. He didn't make Snake Canyon. He didn't make Wembley. He didn't make any of these jumps at all, but he knew, 'If I can just get to the other side alive, I'm gonna be a millionaire.

Like, if I can just get over there somehow and stay alive, I'll be a millionaire.'

There's that insane footage of him coming down the ramp, taking off, flying over all those buses, the bike landing and the suspension compressor throwing him off. He looks like a rag doll that's smashed all over the place.

Then all these rumours started to come out that he broke every single bone in his body, but he still was all right and he was going to do it again! Again! In interviews he always said this: 'Bones heal. Chicks dig scars. Pain is temporary. Glory is forever.'

Now when you were a young fellow, you hear that, you're like, 'I've just been ripped off by a priest for being an altar boy; I got boring dead-behind-the-eyes teachers; my old man, he never talks and he's got a bloody bald patch, but here is *this* crazy guy in his heels and his cape!' Like it was invigorating. Such an amazing thing.

Every time I cycled the bike after I discovered Evel Knievel I was making noises, 'vroom, vroom' noises, and I even asked my da to get me an engine for the pushbike, which I thought was a possibility back then. I was begging him. Please? Please? He'd always say, 'Yeah, yeah, I will, I'll get around to it.'

Why did he say that? *I'll get around to it, I'll get around to it.* Why did he do that? Like just say *No, it can't be done.* Maybe he thought I'd asked for an actual motorbike? I don't know.

'I've ordered it, it's coming, it's coming. Tommy, my friend. Tommy's getting it.'

So, you're looking forward to something that's never going to happen. Like when he told me the southside was Disneyland. We're standing in Clontarf looking at the Poolbeg Towers and Dún Laoghaire, watching people walking around East Wall, and he points and says, 'Disneyland, it's over there.'

'What! Why can't we go!'

'Too far. Cost a fortune. Takes the plane a whole day to get over there.'

We did get to the real Disneyland in the end. In 1984, when I was nine, we went to America. It was the year the Olympics were held in Los Angeles, the one where everyone got done for all the doping. We were off to visit relatives in Arizona, of all places. But we were going to LA first.

I'll never forget being on the jumbo jet. *A JUMBO JET.* Like no one I knew had ever been on a jumbo jet. This was literally a time when people still talked about going to the Continent. If you were rich.

People said 'the Continent' when they meant Spain or France or whatever. No one had been to the States unless they went there on a coffin ship or were going to, like, work illegally and never come home.

And here we were, the Gallaghers, going over to Disneyland on our holidays.

Zsu Zsu from Number 62 came with us. The minute she heard we were going to LA she said, 'Well I'm going with you.' Even me uncle, Fr Traveling Matt, came along for the ride.

This was a time when they used to pull down the screen at the front of the plane, projector style. I was dumbstruck. People were smoking fags and everything. It was brilliant. *Greystoke: The Legend of Tarzan, Lord of the Apes* and *Jaws* were the movies that were showing and I remember watching *Rising Damp*, which, to this day, is still one of my favourite TV shows.

Coming out at the airport there was this big eagle on the

wall, the TSA Eagle I think it was. To me the eagle was like some sort of arch into America.

Disneyland was eventful. The old man collapsed, locked. He was still wearing the same clothes of course, his tweed jackets and Arthur Daley hats and the whole lot. It's 100-degree heat and he's his hat and tie on. Down like a rope. I'm there in my shorts and my Britvic T-shirt and my old man is on the ground foaming at the mouth, drunk and dehydrated within an inch of his life, someone ramming a wallet down his throat. Never worked out what they were doing that for, maybe to open his airways or something? Anyway, he came around eventually but the whole day was ruined.

After Disneyland we went to meet my cousins in Arizona. I don't think most Irish people were aware of Arizona unless they'd seen it in a Clint Eastwood movie. We weren't even in Phoenix, Arizona, we were in Clyde, Arizona, the middle of the desert. The best bit about it was being introduced to all these things that you only ever saw on telly. Brown paper bags for carrying groceries and Dr Pepper and Cherry Coke and watching *The Dukes of Hazzard* while actually in the States. My sister was attacked by red ants. My cousins had names like Dakota and Abigail and Victoria. It all felt so American, like a totally different world.

One morning I woke up and my folks had disappeared in the middle of the night to go to Las Vegas. My dad got his photo taken in the Playboy Club and brought me back an ashtray with a bunny on it and a couple of key rings. I loved that ashtray.

It wasn't long after we got back from America that my granny took the pub off of my da. I don't know the ins and outs, it wasn't something he talked about, but she disinherited him, that's what it boils down to.

The man wasn't capable of doing a good job. He was sick, chronically alcoholic and drinking the business into the ground. But still, to take his livelihood off of him, it was a bastarding thing to do. He never recovered from it.

With whatever money she settled on him they bought a house in Clontarf. And that's when things got really interesting.

5.
Madhouse

Tara died soon after we moved to Clontarf and Joy walked into our lives. Joy was nuts. Where Tara was a lovely, peaceful, playful, loyal, safe dog, Joy was a crazy Labrador. She couldn't sit still for a minute. This thing chewed everything.

She walked in the door and started chewing. A one-dog non-stop chewing machine: shoes, socks, trousers, jackets, furniture, doors. My aul fella left her in the coal shed one day because he was so upset, and she chewed through the door of the coal shed. He built fences to try and keep her in because she was always running away.

She ate through the fences. Twice. Into the neighbours' garden she went, ate their clothesline. Untrainable; pissing and shitting all over the gaff, a wild force of nature. No matter what room you put her in, it got destroyed. So my ma got this black barrel and tied it to her, to slow her down. She chewed her way through a fence and ran away, dragging the barrel behind her. Bonkers.

The last time she ran away my ma, exhausted at this stage, suggested we didn't go looking for her, but I couldn't stick it, so we went looking again but that time we didn't find her. I'd say she took about 100,000 quid's worth of value off that house. We only had her for about a year, but it was a big year in the Gallagher family. That was the year the men arrived.

The house my parents had bought in Clontarf was a big, long bungalow. Having grown up in Marino not far from town, not far from the Ballybough flats, ending up in a big house in leafy Clontarf was a big shift. Everyone thought we were posh and I got slagged over it. But what they didn't realize was that half my house was a mental home.

When my parents bought the house the idea was to take in boarders to help make ends meet. Not just any boarders; these were men who had been in long-term psychiatric care. Psychiatric institutions across the country were closing and these men had nowhere to go, so some of them came and lived in our house. I suppose with my mother's background in nursing, someone, somewhere, thought this was a good idea.

When writing the play *Madhouse* we did some research into how this situation could have happened. How did anyone think this was a good idea? What we discovered was that 'boarding out' was a practice permitted under 1945 mental health legislation. It wasn't very common because there was a legitimate concern that boarded-out patients could be abused or exploited, mainly by being used as cheap labour. Six boarders in a domestic home like ours (being looked after by a woman whose nursing qualification was in her sister's name) was especially unusual. The entire practice ended in the 90s.

At all times there were bona fide mental patients living in one half of our house and we were in the other half. But no one went to the trouble of building a dividing wall. When you went through our front door and turned right, you were in mad land, where the mad lads lived – three bedrooms, two bathrooms and a room where they'd eat and smoke and watch telly. And when you went through the front door and you turned left it was me, Ma, Da, Stacey and the dog.

It seemed like that house was set up to be a madhouse before we even got there. There were the stuffed animals for a start – a deer's head in the hall that terrified me my whole life, and stuffed owls in glass domes. Outside there was a swimming pool with no water in it, and inside a huge fish tank that was only ever half-full because it took so long to fill it.

There was one fish in that giant tank. We called him Christopher Columbus because his world was flat. Talk about a fish putting in a good fight – Christopher enjoyed the madness of that house. He lasted so long that in the end he wasn't gold any more; he'd lost all his colour and turned white, but Christopher held on – he had a lot to live for, that fish.

The boarders who came to live with us, some would have first been admitted to psychiatric hospitals with serious mental illnesses or schizophrenia. However, most were people who at some stage in their lives had developed a small mental health problem – maybe they were depressed, or had a nervous breakdown, or suffered a trauma. Nowadays they'd be given a load of Prozac and someone to talk to, but in the 40s or 50s they were institutionalized, and their small mental health problems developed into big mental illnesses, and they became completely dependent to the point that they couldn't do anything for themselves any more.

Things weren't much better in the 80s and 90s. If you

suffered chronically with depression you took to the bed, that was what people said: 'He took to the bed.' Or if you had an anxiety attack every day, you'd 'trouble with your nerves'. Other than that, you were totally grand.

There still wasn't much talk about 'mental health'; you were still either 'mental', or you had your health. No one wanted to talk about psychiatric illness.

'He's not right in the head, God bless him.'

As if that made anything any better.

'He's in the nip pulling his bleedin' pecker off; he thinks there's a ghost in his head; he thinks he's being chased by a vampire. Don't worry about it though, he's harmless.'

He's harmless. As if the only person he could hurt was himself, so that was all right.

My ma did everything for the men who came to live with us. She sourced their clothes, washed their clothes, made their beds, fed them, and tried to stop them killing each other over what was on the telly. It's amazing how two channels can separate a room. When you've twenty channels there's nothing on, but when there's only two everybody wants to watch one of them. There could be news on one and snooker on the other one. Ructions.

She cut everything off them, all their bits: toenails, fingernails, hair, bits of whatever would be growing out of their ears or their nose. One of the lads thought there was a dog in his stomach, so she'd have to time the snips between barks or she'd stab him in the head. And when he wasn't barking he was talking. Just non-stop chat.

My ma had to do it all. They weren't going to do it, they didn't care how they looked; they were wearing clothes they found in a charity bag, ill-fitting high-waisted trousers and comfortable shoes. They all walked a lot, so every one of them loved a comfortable shoe.

My ma did all the cooking. Any time my da cooked there was war, he burnt the bejaysus out of everything. How? I've started cooking now, do you know how hard it is to burn steel? To burn a pot? It's difficult. He managed to do it every single time he went into the kitchen.

The only time I ever burnt anything was one Christmas. My old man had bought a turkey the size of an ostrich to feed the ten of us in the house and my ma had it all ready in the oven.

'Listen, all I want you to do is turn that knob at 12 o'clock and when I get home it'll be ready.'

I didn't fancy hanging around for a few hours to turn on a bleedin' cooker so the minute she left I turned it on and went out. By the time she got back that turkey was a skeleton.

She kind of saw the funny side, but my old fella was very upset. That turkey had cost him a fortune.

The big job, looking after the men, was administering their pills; these lads were on so many pills, the pills must have been half their problem. The pills were like a starter, a bowl of pills you'd need to tackle with a knife and fork. They'd wash them down with a glass of milk and then they'd get their main course, which was just Mammy food, followed by dessert and cigarettes.

The daily turmoil of getting their medication right. There was a system to the pills and me ma, she learnt it. Six plates, seventy bottles of pills, and she'd just make these little cocktails.

'Two of them, one of them, three of them. Two of those, one of those, six of them. Five of them, two of these, three of those. Four of these, seven of them, one of those and a drink of this.'

It was like watching a wizard at work, or a witch making a broth. Unbelievable.

She'd give it to all the lads, the lads would get sedated, everyone was happy. Three hours or whatever they're all grand, then it's dinner time and it all starts again.

But you think you can do things well? You'd want to have seen her play the pill cabinet. She was like Beethoven playing the piano. Majestic. Whenever she went away and me da was left in charge, you wouldn't know what he'd give them. His patience would run out and he'd just give them pills that looked like they should fit them.

'James looks like he takes blue pills, he's getting the blue pills. Dan, his skin is orange in parts, give him the orange pills.'

With my aul fella in charge there were definitely days they didn't get any pills at all.

6.
The devil and the *Sunday World*

If you've never heard the expression 'house Mass', count yourself lucky. My mother would throw these house Masses all the time. Uncle Matt would be the priest/MC, guzzling the altar wine, and all her sisters and her brothers would come and a load of cousins.

Then the men would be brought in and made to sit down as well. It was just tedious, like there was a perfectly good television turned off while we all engaged in this weird pantomime.

My old fella sat in the same chair every day with his magic can of Guinness. No one ever saw him get up, go to the fridge and sit back down again but there was always Guinness in that can. Every time he picked it up it was half full. There was always only ever one can, you'd never see cans in the kitchen or in the bin, just this one can that he could constantly pour. To this day I have no idea how he did it.

He'd go fairly heavy on the can during the house Mass because he didn't want to be there, none of us did. Most of the time he'd pass out as soon as it started, snoring and groaning. It was a bit of craic and he'd keep it low level enough. Occasionally my ma would turn around and shush him and the Mass would go on.

But on one memorable occasion when Uncle Matt raised the chalice in the middle of proceedings, my da woke up with a start, jumped out of his chair and shouted, 'Wahey, thanks be to Jesus.' He ran behind the altar, lifted up the chalice, banged it down on the table and started yelling, 'Halle-fucking-lujah!' We were roaring laughing at this stage, like it's gone, Mass is gone, all the old ones with their mouths falling open, and him just singing, 'Hallelujah. Praise be to Holy Jesus.'

Then he sat back down, cackled away to himself and passed out. Straight asleep as if someone just turned him off. As if someone had flicked a switch on his neck and cut the power. Head just dropped. He'd ruined everything but it was a glorious moment.

Jesus was around an awful lot when I was young – he was very hard to get away from.

My da's sister Eileen and my ma never really got on, but they did have Jesus and Mary in common. We'd go down to Cork on our holidays most years, and I'd be bored out of my mind. There was nothing to do but eat Silvermints, look at cows.

One year in the middle of all this monotony Auntie Eileen said we were going somewhere exciting. Immediately I'm thinking Trabolgan, right? My cousin Tadhg had told me all about it, that it had a wave machine in the pool like a tsunami. In retrospect I should have known not to listen to Tadhg; this is a lad who was up in Dublin with us once, went on a double-decker bus and thought it was a rollercoaster.

Hours of driving and we finally arrived at this place with a big tent, but straight away as a young fella I knew something was off because there were no food stalls and no rides. Even when you went to the horse racing as a kid there'd be merry-go-rounds. There was none of that.

The place was full of priests with guitars and aul ones in headscarves with that aul one print that you never see any more, a brown sort of tartan. Now I say aul ones, they were probably thirty-two, but they were ageing quickly with a scatter of kids and maybe a bald husband in tow.

It wasn't like Mass. It wasn't the usual 'boredidy boredidy boredidy, this Jesus fella's dead and it's all your fault'. It wasn't that. Instead, it was like a party for a ninety-five-year-old in a tent that 700 people had turned up to. All these people in a tent carrying on like it was Jesus's ninety-fifth birthday and that Jesus was there!

'Hello, Jesus, how are you? Are you delighted? Are you delighted, Jesus, that we're all here? Oh my God. I can't believe all these people have come to see you, Jesus.'

Every so often someone would scream, 'Does anybody feel the JEEEESUUUUS in the room?'

Then all the aul ones would start going 'bappity, bappity, boppiby boo, gobbidy, goddiby goo', channelling Jesus. As if Jesus was going to talk through a thirty-six-year-old woman with a Tullamore accent. As if that's how Jesus would bring himself into the world, that's how Jesus was going to send us a message: 'Offaly, offaly, offaly.'

They got to the sign of peace and as a young fella I put my hand down straight away, I wasn't shaking hands with any of these lunatics, but total strangers just wrapped their arms around me. At Camp Jesus the sign of peace was a full-on hug. There was this weird euphoria in the tent, everyone crying and hugging each other while the priest was up on stage singing, 'Mary had a baby, oh my Lord.

Mary had a baby. Oh Lord. People keep a'coming but the train done gone.'

It was overwhelming. In the car on the way home my cousins had a tape of all the Jesus songs, and they knew all the words, singing their hearts out about Jesus's love.

'It's so high you can't get over it, so low you can't get under it, so wide you can't get round it, oh wonderful love.'

Hours of it. There were no motorways, so at the time a day trip from Cork city to Clonakilty took about two days. At least, it felt like two days.

I'll never ever forget the madness, then getting home and me old fella saying, 'How was it?' and me saying, 'Well, it wasn't bleedin' Trabolgan.'

In my head I remember Camp Jesus being about a week long, but I don't remember any nights there so it's possible it was one long day. The whole thing had a strange effect on me. After it I was so alert and aware of all the Jesus shenanigans going on around me. That was the year the statues started moving and dancing down in Ballinspittle and all over Ireland. 1985.

My Auntie Eileen loved nothing more than a moving statue.

'I was there all day, right? And the sun splitting the stones, right? The heat FIT to kill you. And I was looking at a statue, riiiiiight? And I swear to God, the sun started dancing in the sky.'

Course it did! You're massively dehydrated in July standing there looking at a statue with thousands of other lunatics.

Then the three of them, Ma, Auntie Eileen and Ma's friend Fr Mick Maher, went off to Medjugorje in the old Yugoslavia, behind the Iron Curtain, for two weeks to see the children who had communed with the Virgin Mary.

Off they went to the Virgin Mary gig. The thing about the

Virgin Mary gig, though, is you never got to see the gig itself, you only got to see the audience of children who'd been at it.

Meanwhile, back in Clontarf, Da fed me and Stacey chocolate yogurts and pizza slices for two weeks. Fantastic.

The only religion I really got into was through Fr Maher. He wasn't really into God or Jesus or any of the disciples. He was just mad into the devil. Like he was MAD into the devil. So he was very interesting because he was kind of like telling you the boogeyman stories.

Everyone was always saying that God was everywhere. He's sitting in the chair, he's in your ma's hair, there were all these songs about God being everywhere. Mick was the opposite.

'Oh, the devil, you have to be careful – the devil's in your dinner, the devil's in your boots, the devil's in your music, the devil's in your shoes. He dresses up and he looks like people and he's always trying to influence you to do mad stuff. He gets into your dreams and he gives you thoughts and temptations. He gives you choices and you'll always take the devil's choice but he'll make you *think* that you thought of it yourself.'

It was brilliant stuff. He gave me a sticker of the prayer to the Archangel Michael and I stuck it on the end of my bed. This was my defence against the devil. Now I can't remember the Hail Mary, the Glory Be or the Rosary, none of that. But I remember that prayer.

'Blessed Michael Archangel, defend us in our hour of conflict, be our safeguard against the wickedness and snares of the devil and may God restrain him. We humbly pray.'

There's four verses to that thing and I can get all the way to the bottom.

On the sticker there was an image of the Archangel Michael standing on the devil's head on a rock with a big sword. Now, this was the type of religion I could get into; this was Action Man Angel shit.

Fr Mick would talk a lot about the time he went to the Holy Hill in Medjugorje with me ma. He said even on Holy Hill, the Devil would get people, whispering all kinds of dirt and lies to them. 'Don't believe them bitches,' he'd whisper into your ear, 'they're only telling you lies. They never saw the Virgin Mary at all!'

That was the big thing with Fr Mick: whatever you do, do not listen to the Devil. He's an absolute bastard.

The thing is I did believe in God, right up until quite late in life for all the good it did me, but even as a young fellow, I never really bought into all the rigmarole. In Belgrove they used to do confession, there would be days where they set up these little fold-up confession boxes, and you had to go in and tell the priest your sins.

I always thought this was just weird and so did the lads in my class. You could always see the lads' feet dangling at the bottom of the box, so we made up a load of foot signals. You tapped your foot up and down when things were going all right, but if you moved your foot on the heel side to side it meant, 'I'm a bit freaked out by this fella now.'

If you lifted up your heel and you tapped your heel up and down, it just meant you were doing the usual: 'I called me ma a bitch and stole a fiver out of her pocket and told lots of lies and didn't do the cleaning up.'

So, you could look at all the feet and know what was going on, which is always a bit of an adventure, and you'd be looking for the fellow who was spinning on his heel 'cause you knew that priest would be easier on you, stick you with less penance to do. (How do they work that out, by the way? Like how do they work out the price for the sin? Is there a list? Sentencing guidelines, like in the courts?)

Wouldn't you love to just go back and do it now, though? Go to confession but tell the truth. Sit in that box as a twelve-year-old and say, 'I smoked a John Player Blue and had a wank.'

People get outraged now because of everything that's come out about the church. But even as young people in the 80s we knew the priests were talking shite when they were giving us sex education.

'You have to love each other . . . daddy and mammy have a special cuddle . . . if you touch your mickey hair will grow out of your ears.'

Somehow, they were the guiding hand of Irish sexual lives. No wonder we needed six pints of Brewmaster to even rub our goolies off each other. I mean, you were coming out of the closet just admitting you'd any sexual desire at all.

Course it was different when they were doing it. Then it was: *Poor Fr Michael had a moment of weakness.* You're the one who should have known better, a dirty sinner. Not the fella who promised to be celibate for the glory of God.

The first time I rubbed one out, it was a page with a set of tits on it, and my ma caught me with it in my back pocket.

If you wanted to find some dirty magazines, you went down to the train stations. You walked up the tracks a bit on a Sunday and you'd find some in the bushes, torn up. Lads buying them in Belfast and having a wank in the loos. The sixty-mile-an-hour club. Then throwing them out the window when they get to Killester.

So this time I picked up a copy of the *Sunday World* and pulled a page out of it.

I was so lucky that it was on the flip side of the cartoons for kids, because when my ma found it in my pocket, she said:

'I want to have a chat with you.'

'What?'

'Is that a picture of a woman with her tits out?'

Aw, God.

'Yeah, it is, but look, Henry! He's on the back, isn't he?'

She checked and he was. Henry saved me from so much trouble.

The whole experience scared me, but it was brilliant. I was sitting in my room with the picture of the woman and I couldn't wait. I had this horn going and I'm thinking it's either gonna fall off or explode. Oh, it was raging, raging horn, and I didn't know how to really wank. I was just sort of rubbing it. So, I had my mickey in my hand and I'm pulling, doing lines with my fingers. I'm going, 'Whoo,' and looking at the picture every so often.

Oh man, I just couldn't understand the feelings that were going through my head. My heart was racing, and my flute was raging. And then, without even touching it, stuff just flew out of it across the room in one big squirt. I started panicking, I was terrified, thinking, 'Is that cancer? Like, is that cancer inside me, this white goo stuff?'

I remember lying down in bed thinking, 'I'm really sick. I'm actually really sick. Oh, man. Oh, Jesus. How am I gonna tell my ma to take me to the doctor? I'm gonna go to the doctor and what am I gonna tell the doctor?'

On and on in my head until, of course, an hour later I'm like, *Let's have a look at that picture again.*

7.
Moolah

You know the way some people are naturally singers and some people are naturally dancers and some people are naturally painters? Well, some people are naturally entrepreneurs. It's a talent in the exact same way, a natural-born gift.

Being an entrepreneur is an art and it deserves tax exemption because an entrepreneur has to rearrange the world.

There was a young entrepreneur in our class in Belgrove. At break we used to play a game that involved a window ledge: if you got your ass on that ledge you were safe, you couldn't be hit. But because it was a window ledge there was a pane of glass. So, one day one of the lads was running, running, running and he jumped to get his ass on the ledge. He's flying through the air and goes through the window. Incredibly, he wasn't cut but we were all hauled up to the principal's office.

'What happened?'

'I was chasing him.'

'You were chasing him, were you?'

Why do teachers do that, make you feel small by repeating everything you say straight back to you?

Yeah. I was chasing him and he jumped in the air.

He jumped in the air?

And he was flying backwards.

He was flying backwards?

And his arse went through the glass.

His arse went through the glass?

Yes! This is what I'm telling you, you gobshite!

When this happened we were in the last year of primary school, sixth class, so at the most we're twelve years old. It was fifteen pounds to replace that window, which was a total lie because glass was not expensive in the 80s.

The principal was giving us all, 'Where are your parents going to get fifteen pounds to fix that glass?' and the rest of it when this young fella puts his hand in his pocket, takes out a bundle of pound notes and goes:

'1, 2, 3, 4, 5, 1, 2, 3, 4, 5, 1, 2, 3, 4, 5.'

Now the principal is in a state of shock, he wasn't expecting that. He gets the parents on the phone immediately and says, 'D'you know your son is walking around with about sixty pounds in the pocket of his O'Neill shorts?'

'We know, we can't stop him working. He's been cutting grass for all the neighbours. He's been saving up all his money. He's got hundreds of pounds. Hundreds.'

Most of us get to a point, you know, when we're thirty-five and think *I'm gonna read Trump's book and learn how to be a millionaire, or Branson's autobiography, see how he did it.* But it's an impossible skill to learn, it's a natural-born given talent. And that young fella had it in spades.

*

Money has freaked me out my WHOLE life. My folks were always panicking about it and me aul fella would spend it like there was no tomorrow. Any time the accountant was coming around me da was in bits over it and he'd never open his post because they were all bills.

Even as a young fellow I'd be saying, 'Would you just open the bleedin' things?' 'Will you talk to someone about it?'

Ignore them and they'll go away seemed to be the method always employed. And that just does not work. The house in Clontarf was always in jeopardy. So much anxiety built up in the house about losing the house – losing everything – that everyone was in a blind panic all of the time.

That's why when I did make a few quid for the first time in my life I finally felt a bit of stability and came to the conclusion that money is the way out. The only way out. No matter what anyone says, money matters. Money is freedom.

If you have money you've better healthcare, better holidays, better everything. If I didn't have a few quid to pay me health insurance, I wouldn't have gotten into St Pat's, and I'd be dead now.

Don't listen to the people who say money isn't everything. It is everything. And everything that is not money is completely disposable. You have to swap your time for money because you don't get either of them back.

No matter how much money you have, somebody wants it, so you have to have too much, to keep some for yourself. And the great thing as well is, if you don't want someone in your life, give them money.

'D'you want a loan of a few quid?'

'Yeah.'

You'll never see them again.

Friends come and go, experiences come and go, but every

second you're running out of money and time and one day you'll be dead. It's only people in the first world who would ever say money isn't important.

In the 80s you were encouraged to have a job by the time you were twelve, but it was really hard to make a few quid. My first job was delivering leaflets for Nolan's Supermarket. They gave you a little map, and with these little fluorescent markers they would highlight the streets where they wanted you to put the leaflets through the doors. I can't remember what they paid us, but I do remember it was not good – one penny a leaflet or something like that. My friend Peter got me into it, but I didn't have the patience. After a few streets I'd just put them in the postbox and go home. Or stack them up in the garage and they'd be grand there. My reckoning was, 'If somebody finds them in ten years, they're not gonna sue me for the 3.99 I illegally claimed from Clontarf's Food Superstore the few weeks I worked there.'

Nolan's is an institution and is still going strong. And no wonder, the prices they charge. It's the Brown Thomas of cabbage: it's that expensive, I don't know how you don't come out wearing the vegetables, to be honest with you. Still, much as I slag them I shop there all the time. One day on Nova I was slagging them, saying you couldn't buy one thing in their shop for two euro. A few days later me and Kelly were in. By the time we got to the checkout they'd made us up a big hamper full of everything they sell for two euro, from pasta sauces and capers to chocolate and raisins. They got the last laugh. And we got a brilliant hamper.

My ma was a big fan of Nolan's. For years she had my credit card in her purse, and I'd be overdrawn wondering how the hell that happened. When I'd look at my statement

I'd see she'd bought a washing machine and a jacuzzi. So I gave her a Revolut card; it was easier to track her spending with a Revolut card.

In lockdown my phone would ping and there she'd be in Nolan's paying 37 euro for an onion. Why couldn't she go to Lidl, it would have been a hell of a lot cheaper. We were back in Marino nearly fifteen years at this stage but she still went to Nolan's of Clontarf for her groceries.

I suppose, in fairness to her, her weekly trip to Nolan's was the only time she left the house; it was her social outlet, promenading down the aisles of potatoes and leeks.

My God, was she a ferocious snob. And she'd absolutely no right to be.

'Don't be going down there now to Marino.'

'Wha'?'

'You wouldn't like it, the people who live there.'

'What are you talking about? That's where we live! That's where we're from!'

'Oh! Don't be telling that to people!'

'This is bleedin' Marino! To get to Clontarf you have to go under the bridge and on to the seafront, it's not far but –'

'Well, I prefer to go to Nolan's. People behave better in Clontarf.'

A mad woman. A thundering, thundering snob.

8.

'Where's your maniacs?'

Most of the men used to leave the house during the day, go for walks or down to the day centre for a cup of milk and a bun, play draughts and smoke more cigarettes. For some reason there's a real correlation between how mad you are and the amount of cigarettes you smoke. I've seen enough mental patients in my life to know how much of a truth that is. The further your mind goes away and gets lost, the more you smoke, and when the mind has gone completely you just chain-smoke all day long; it's an unbroken passion for nicotine.

When we were selling the house in Clontarf years later, I remember painting the room that they smoked in and I swear to God, it must've been fifty coats of paint I put on it, and you still couldn't get rid of the smell of smoke.

My da spent as much time as he could out of that house. The pub was only 200 yards down the road but he refused to walk to it and it would drive the neighbours mad, him cruising along at twelve miles per hour in the Bluebird. That's what he called his car; he loved it, but it was an ancient old banger of a thing.

On Sundays he was made to take the men to Mass. It was some sight, my da with four or five of the lads crammed in the back of the Bluebird, smoke pouring out of every window. He'd drop them at the church, rob the Mass leaflet to show me ma later and head down to the Sheds for a few pints. Then he'd forget all about the lads and they'd have to find their own way home.

Most of the men were elderly by the time they came to live with us, and even at a young age it's strange how you get used to things. Watching *Home and Away* one day after school, I heard the sound of someone hitting the deck. When I went for a look, I found one of the men lying with his hands down by his sides and blood on the outside of the bath. He never really recovered from that fall and died soon after.

A few of the men died in the house. Many weren't in great health when they arrived, and were in and out of the hospital a fair bit. You got used to arriving home from school and seeing an ambulance outside the gaff and wondering who it was for.

Everyone was in a constant state of high alert when James arrived, he had this unbelievable thirst for tap water. And it was serious – he could have died from water intoxication, that's a real thing! – so you had to watch him like a hawk around the taps. The pills were the only thing that stopped him from overdosing, probably because after a load of them he couldn't even remember what water was.

Another of the men got into the bath one day and turned over in it. He just took a whim and said to himself, 'Do you know what would be good? If I turn around in the bath, face down.'

He didn't want to drown; we could hear him trying hard to get himself back facing the right way again. My mother had to shove me through the bathroom window because the door was locked. When I got in his back was arched. I opened the door and my mother pulled him out.

She was always great in an emergency like that. But then, if you had to stand on a chair to change a light bulb, she could go to a point of full hysteria.

'You're going to fall. Ahh, Jesus. The glass is going to break and smash into your eyes, you're going to be blind. *You're going to be blind!'*

The whole house would be up the wall over the smallest thing. Barking dog, shaking legs, distressed children, upset neighbours. All over a light bulb. But your man nearly drowning in the bath behind a locked door? No problem.

She always seemed to react to things in the exact opposite way most people did. For instance, when one of the men joined the Workers' Party she thought it was the weirdest thing any of them had ever done, and it really, really wasn't.

Someone would come up to me and say, 'Do you ever see your man hiding behind trees and chasing squirrels in the park?'

'Yeah, I live with him, I know him well, I made him a tuna sandwich yesterday. I can tell you what his tablets are. They don't seem to have much of an effect, but we keep piling them in.'

People behaving crazily, for want of a better word, has never bothered me the same way it bothers other people. Recently I was in a café, and there was a woman staring through the window at people eating their food. When I looked up from a bite she caught my eye and started roaring at me, 'Fuck off you, you fucking fucker.'

Everyone was stressed but I was like, 'It's grand, it's fine, it gives her a little bit of relief.' I was genuinely delighted for her.

One of the men used to think a fellow called Barney was trying to kill him. My ma told me Barney was some lad that was in one of the homes he was in before who must have beaten him or something. The poor man was terrified of Barney coming for him, it was a real paranoia.

Another fella wore black all the time and used to go for the longest walks. He'd say he was off for a walk at 7pm and he'd come back Tuesday.

The most disturbed man who lived with us thought everyone was following him all the time. He was tormented, that lad. It would take him so long to cross the road: looking behind trees, at the top of the stairs, you'd see his head appear and disappear constantly. It was hypnotic to watch him, it really was, bobbing around, bobbing and weaving. How he didn't make himself seasick, I don't know.

Every so often he'd go to an off-licence and get locked if he had money for a few cans and then he'd go missing. The rest of the time he'd spend doing laps of the garden.

One fella, much younger than the others, always wore black slacks and a white shirt. He went out for a walk one day and hanged himself from a tree at St David's School. My mother told me that something bad had happened to him there.

There were always six patients and a revolving door. Many faces came and went, male faces. There was one woman and I've always wondered why she was there. She was functional, she'd do normal things like go out for a meal and I think she even had a job at one stage. She was so much more together than the other lads. What she must have thought going back into that house every day.

*

It was only when I went into other people's homes that I'd really register the differences between their lives and mine. To me a private home was weird and sharing it with six mental patients was normal. Those houses were too quiet, just had family in them. They'd be eating dinner, watching TV, and I'd be thinking, 'Where's your maniacs? Did they get out? You better look for them! I'm sure it's time for their pills and cigarettes!'

People talk about farmers never having a day off; you have to feed the cattle and feed the sheep and the goats, plant the crops and plant the seeds and no matter what the weather, you have to go out into it. Fair enough. But try looking after people with serious psychiatric problems, people who you might have to spend the day looking for because they went for an extremely long walk the night before and got lost and didn't come home.

Give me crops and cattle any day over an invisible gorilla and the lad who's trying to run away from it, or a guy who thinks there's a dog in his stomach or a fella who thinks the IRA are after him so he keeps running up into the attic. My ma dealt with that kind of craic morning, noon and night, as well as washing their clothes, cutting their hair and at the same time making them food. Meanwhile my da was in the pub or watching Sally Jessy Raphael in the front room, drinking his magic can of Guinness and pretending to hoover.

When that's your day-to-day you don't know what normal is, you're totally out of touch with it. You forget that people live with just their families. You forget that your house is not like their house.

If you had people coming in some man might walk by them looking over his shoulder or barking like a dog.

'Who's that?'

Long story.

At first you don't know how to explain the six men walking around because you don't know what's going on yourself.

Then, when you've worked it out, you're too embarrassed to explain it and then after a while you're so accustomed to it you don't explain it at all.

It never dawned on me until much later that everyone assumed these men were my family. People would ask me were they my uncles or my da's mates. *His mates? What are you talking about?*

Because the thing is I thought this was happening all over the country. It really did take me a while to work out how weird it was.

You tell people, 'I grew up in a madhouse,' and everyone goes, 'Haha, didn't we all?'

And I'm like, 'No, no, an actual madhouse, full of mentally ill people.' And they can't believe it and I don't blame them.

There had to be a million easier ways to make money. A million ways. It's not as if my ma was even that well paid, she was still coming back from the supermarket with yellow pack cornflakes, she still had ten mouths to feed on those wages. And a dog.

Then you watch shows like *The Brady Bunch* on TV or *The Waltons*. Those shows were very hard to swallow. They might as well have been science fiction. Big happy families? All going to bed and saying Goodnight to each other? Bananas. Life in our house was such a mad, mad, mad experience.

Nobody really knew anyone else because everyone was so busy except for me da; the men flat-out smoking, my ma run off her feet and my sister doing whatever it was she was doing.

My main focus was to do everything I could to not be in the house, to get out and about. Family? I didn't know my family any better than I knew the lads in the house. It's only as we're getting older that my relationship with Stacey is really starting to develop, because there was no family life when we were kids, at all.

There's no way you're coming out of that environment and getting into law school or studying medicine. That's not going to happen. Your sense of reality is completely warped. And the men being in the house wasn't even the main problem. The big problem was the booze.

One of the reasons I wouldn't go into a psychiatric Institution – like one of the main reasons – was because I thought it would be like the home I grew up in. I thought mental hospitals were full of people who never get their brain back. And I mean 'brain', not 'mind', like a part of your actual physical brain is removed. That's how I understood the people who came to live with us in the house – it was like part of their brain had been removed, that's how damaged they seemed to me.

My experience of former psychiatric patients was of people thinking there was a Jack Russell in their belly, people who kept thousands of pounds wrapped up in the lining of their coat, people who went on walks and got lost for three days, people who talked to imaginary gorillas, people hiding in hedges. The man hiding in the hedge – I don't know if he thought he was being followed by the IRA or the CIA or the INLA or the RNLI, but he was terrified.

I grew up in a psychiatric experiment crossed with an alcoholic experiment. That's probably what most people would have said it was, you know, from the outside looking in: 'Oh, that's the place with the mentallers and the drunks in it.' It was a place run by two people who were extraordinarily drunk and guarded by a potentially vicious dog with a brain tumour.

9.
Huggy Bear

By now you know how much I love dogs – usually, they were the only bit of sanity in the house (apart from Stacey, who was too young to count). But Skippy was a special case, he actually *chose* to come and live with us.

Skippy arrived that time I was down at Camp Jesus. My ma rang me from Dublin and said, 'You won't believe it, the most beautiful dog has just walked into the house.'

Skippy turned up one day out of the blue and refused to leave. He was an absolute head-turner. A rough collie, like Lassie, but white with two brown patches over his ears and down into his eyes. An unbelievably good-looking dog. Trying to be cool as a teenager I would be a bit embarrassed because he was so flamboyant, he properly demanded attention. Cars would slow down to look at him. It was like going for a walk with Danny La Rue.

The only problem was he didn't like other dogs, he only liked us. He didn't even like his original owners. We brought him back to them a couple of times and he wasn't having it.

Eventually they said, 'Look, keep him, he obviously doesn't like us any more.' Which is pretty un-doglike behaviour. You know there's something wrong with you if your dog walks out on you. A wife can leave anybody, a husband can leave anybody, cats will leave you at the first sniff of a better offer. But a dog? How can you look at yourself and think, 'That wasn't my fault.' It definitely was. I don't know how you get over that. Granted, Joy did leave us but that was because she wasn't the full shilling, the poor dog was demented. Skippy just couldn't stand his owners and somehow thought it was better in our house, even though it was absolutely chaotic in every way.

Poor Skippy got a brain tumour in the end, he'd get sudden pains in his head and think you were attacking him and then he'd attack you. That was the end of him. That was very sad. Me ma rang me and said, 'He's gone.' Out of nowhere.

When I went into St Pat's I thought it was going to be something along the lines of what I grew up with, just on a grand scale where the only normal person would be a five-year-old girl called Stacey. I don't know if I envisaged drunk nurses feeding us or arranging our tablets by colour according to our height or whatever, like me aul fella would do when he was left in charge, but I fought going into that place so much.

There was just this wildness in the house when we were kids and you never had any idea what was going on, ever. And more than that, you didn't want to know. Your one thought the whole time was 'Let's get out of this crazy place.'

Someone asked me once, did I ever feel nervous? Nervous?

Nervous? I was fucking shitting meself. But not because of the men, I was shitting myself all the time wondering what might happen next, you know?

It's like when they say to working-class lads, 'Oh, you probably grew up tough, did you?' And it's like, no, I was just worried the whole time. Worried every day that some lunatic was going to batter me.

In our house it was more like, *What am I walking into?* Literally from one minute to the next you'd be thinking this. All this going on the whole time and me just being this mad lost young boy in it all, living in this mad environment, this mental environment where you can't sit still for a second and you don't know what's going to happen next.

Then you go to school and you have to sit down for five hours and listen to someone banging on about Jesus or Irish or maths.

'I can't sit down. Are you out of your mind? How am I supposed to sit down? I've never done that.'

Then you're called disruptive. So, you don't – you CAN'T – fit in. You don't fit in at school and you don't fit in at home and you don't fit in anywhere and you don't have anywhere to really go. So you think, well, at least if I aim for being bad, I have some sort of a title, you know?

If people tell you you're bad often enough you think, right, I'll live up to it, at least it's some sort of an identity. And I was a bollox.

When I was five or six I witnessed boldness for boldness's sake for the first time ever and it was a joyous experience, something that made a real, lasting impression on me. My folks must have been tired of having me underfoot all day at the pub because they hauled me off to a northside institution, Billie Barry's Stage School. Same as with my Communion, I'd very little say in the matter.

'You're gonna do something new.'

'What is it?'

'Just get in the car.'

We drove around to Fairview Parish Hall and when I went in at the back of the hall there's this big aul one playing the piano. Then another aul one – Billie Barry herself – started lashing instructions at us.

'Tap with the right foot and stop!'

'And tap with the left foot and stop!'

We're all there doing what we were told in our little lines when a young fella started running up and down the hall using his tap shoes as skates on the wooden floor. They were roaring at him, 'Stop! Get into the line!'

He wasn't getting into the line.

He was even younger and smaller than me, and he wasn't getting into any line.

Running up and down, running, skating, twisting, jumping on his back, doing little turns. I couldn't believe it.

Billie Barry was like, 'You! You are going to be in a lot of trouble. What's your name?'

And he just looked at her, pointed his finger up at her face and went, 'My name is Huggy Bear!'

Everybody fell around laughing. Even the old crow playing the piano cracked a smile.

That was the first time I ever saw deliberate bad behaviour. That kid hadn't drunk one too many Coca-Colas; he just didn't care. The absolute rebellion of it.

'My name is Huggy Bear! I came here to go sliding. I want to go sliding.'

I was still very young and hadn't fully grasped the concept of misbehaviour yet, but it was a defining moment for sure.*

So I was bold. I was definitely bold. It mostly went unnoticed at home because my parents and the men were bolder. But at school I was one of the worst. I was in trouble all the time.

I was constantly mitching, going missing in the park. When we were eleven, me and my mate Brian, we filled up a cycling bottle with whiskey and orange juice and didn't go to school. Brian was always mad into bikes, even as a kid.

We walked past the school and even waved at the teachers on their way in. Then we sat in a bin shed in Clontarf, drank the whiskey and orange juice. When we left the bin shed, we were officially missing people, the whole place was out looking for us and we just strolled up to the school like nothing had happened. I don't know what convinced us to just return to school, but I'm sure it was lunchtime; we were probably hungry.

This is how I know I'll never be an alcoholic, because I gave it my best shot and failed miserably. Eleven was the age me and my friends started experimenting with booze, and by fifteen we were really well practised at it and drinking in pubs. But I'm a terrible drinker, I can't have a drink when I'm in a bad mood, which is literally the point of drinking if you're an alcoholic.

To this day one of my proudest memories of primary school was when I turned down a gold card. One of our teachers would hand them out for different projects, a 'Well

* I went back to Billie Barry's only a few more times. It was absolute torture because I have no coordination whatsoever. You'll never see me on *Dancing with the Stars*.

done, you' award. I wrote a story and I knew it was good and she gave me a double gold card. She never gave anyone a double gold card. She was incentivizing me. *Finally he's making an effort.*

When I told her I didn't want it you should have seen how furious she was; she called me a cheeky bastard and everything. Oh, I still relish that. Everyone heard me reject it and her whole reward system instantly fell apart. It meant nothing. Now it wasn't a gold card reward system; it was a yellow sticker not worth the paper it was printed on.

You have to understand: this was the same wagon who made me cry when I couldn't work out a sum on the board a few months earlier. When I was trying to do something that was hard for me she threw it back in my face. The essay was easy for me so I threw it back in her face.

All the way through school, as soon as I would see a teacher, I would feel physically ill at the thought of having to be quiet. Like, physically ill. It just got worse in secondary school. Wearing school uniforms and having to sit through mind-numbing bollox. Being told to sit down and think. My body just does not work like that.

Sit down, be quiet, and think.

I just couldn't do it. I'd be looking around at all the other freaks who somehow could and feeling totally inadequate. And then I'd go from there back to the madhouse every day.

10.
Booze

'I would do anything for you.' That's what my ma would always say. 'Anything at all.' To a large extent that was true. She would bend over backwards, give you all her money, sacrifice everything she had for you, stay at home 24/7 and work herself to bits minding six seriously ill men. All of that. But when you said, 'The only thing I want is for you to give up the booze,' she'd just say, 'No, the booze is all I have, it's the one thing that helps me.' This conversation was going on between us as long as I can remember, from a very young age.

So, unfortunately, we were always second best to the bottle. And that was always the most hurtful thing, being second best.

It was the same with my aul man. The two of them lied about it all the time and I've never understood why. I mean, there was no need to lie about their drinking. It wasn't exactly difficult to work out when they were drinking because it was every day.

You can see the change in people when they get drunk, and when you're around people who drink long enough, you can tell if they've just sniffed it. I know it sounds bananas, but you can tell the second it touches their lips. It's a weird thing because other people can't see it as clearly as you can.

'Well, they seem the same to me.'

'I'm telling you, they're pissed.'

People would come and do check-ups on the experiment every so often. Once a year maybe these professional people would turn up, sit down, have a cup of tea and a slice of cake, and head on their way. It wasn't exactly a thorough thing – two hours maybe before the drinking's going to start again and the pill wizardry is back on. I wouldn't be there; I'd be outside setting fires to bins or whatever. The dog would be asleep.

These 'experts' just had this amazing ability to walk in and do their check-up during the calm. An hour after they left the whole place would be going *ding, ding, ding, ding, ding, ding, ding* and turn into a funfair. They'd no idea how mad the place actually was.

When you spend essentially a lot of your life saying to your parents, *This is the one thing I don't want you to do* and they ignore that or, worse, throw it back in your face, then you end up feeling neglected because the reaction was often really, really aggressive.

'Don't you fucking tell me what to do. What the fuck are you talking about? I'm not fucking drinking.'

But you could smell it. They always drank it out of cups or mugs, whiskey mixed with all kinds of weird stuff. Really cheap nasty whiskey, Vat 69, that was the poison that was in the house all the time. And it's pretty hard to disguise a cup or a mug of whiskey. Every dog in north Dublin could smell a cup of whiskey and two kids could smell it too. To have someone standing there holding a teacup or a coffee cup of whiskey and denying it, you're just like, 'You're a fucking liar.'

Telling an addict they're lying is bad news. They get very defensive and very angry. That's the big problem, it just becomes impossible for them to tell the truth. It was confusing as well because the one thing my ma would always say is, 'I hate lies. No matter what it is. Tell me the truth, tell me the truth, tell me the truth.'

'Okay. Are you drinking?'

'No.'

'Right. Fair enough.'

Most of the time I wouldn't say anything but then I'd let myself down, say, 'Don't drink.' Or hide the drink. And the world would turn upside down because they didn't think drinking was the problem, they thought it was the solution. The way they saw it was that they had this one thing to hold on to and enjoy and I was trying to take it off them. They were just doing their thing and I was the one making it worse.

That was when everything got properly nasty and they'd say *You're not our kid* and we'd be killing each other, bringing the house down, mayhem.

Sometimes I just went spare in my head; I'd punch myself in the face as hard as I could. Box myself in the head proper, angry at myself for being angry about something I couldn't do anything about. When I'd no anger left, and nothing left to smash, I'd hide it in myself. I learnt how to turn my anger on and off like a light switch.

The next day no one would say a thing, every day was a new start and by lunchtime the clouds would be forming. There was no day off. It was a never-ending circle of madness.

Sometimes one of their family would take me aside: 'How

are you doing? Are they drinking a lot? Are they really bad? All they have is the bottle, God love them. Well, we need to do something about this.'

Two weeks later the same people are over in the house with bottles of wine, getting drunk. Pack of liars. Calling me up a few days later, giving out about my parents causing trouble, saying they didn't like it. But it was all right for me and Stacey to live there.

I was a chronic bed-wetter until I don't know what age, but whatever age it was I was far too old to be still at that caper. I don't know what it is about the human body that it takes all your trauma and projects it out your pee-hole in your sleep, but it's a hell of a trick.

You try to keep your friends out of your house because you're ashamed of the drinking that goes on. Growing up I didn't resent the people around me who had normal lives. I don't think I resented them, anyway. But I definitely felt shame.

I was ashamed if they turned up in a state to the school or to the local disco nights or whatever was going on. The supermarket was the epicentre of shame. My ma would take me shopping with her and it was brutal, with her falling all over the place. It was so obvious she was drunk. To this day going to the supermarket stresses me out so much I need to pee the minute I walk into one. In restaurants she'd get thick with the staff. It was all just so very, very shameful.

You don't go to drunk parents with your problems because you don't know how they'll react. Maybe they'll turn up at your school plastered and make a holy show of you. Because one thing drunk people are bastards for doing is turning up at things. Drunk people go everywhere. I'd go to big efforts to hide parent-teacher meetings from them, but they'd turn up. Then arrive home and say, 'I got away with that. That was grand.'

They didn't get away with it. They'd been unbelievably out-of-their-minds drunk.

Life was so unpredictable at home, so what happened was I started trusting strangers, like literal strangers. People I'd never met before in my life I trusted more than my own parents, and I don't think that's a good thing for a young person.

11.

Best year ever

When we were doing our Inter Cert the big laugh was 'Imagine you had to do Syllabus C Maths.' Syllabus C Maths is more or less 'How many fingers do you have?' I failed it.

At school it was obvious I had a problem with numbers from the start. I've never done the assessment, but I have dyscalculia. A teacher at St Paul's pointed it out to me, although the word he used was innumerate.

Having no mathematical ability at all has always made me feel terrible because it made me think that I was never going to do anything with my life. Back then, in the dark ages, no matter what you wanted to do you always seemed to need maths and I had no ability to take it in at all.

They put me in a class with a load of others like me. The delight when you met someone who was just as bad at everything as you were. Jesus, you'd have wanted to have seen the state of us. Me, I look like a potato with wonky eyes, or a balloon with a smile drawn on it. And then there was a lad in the class who had the body of a sixty-three-year-old man. He had a big hairy daddy mickey when everyone else was still bald down there.

There were lads in that class who couldn't hold bowls properly or plates or knives and forks, literally headcase young fellas were in that class. Our class was an institution within an institution, a place they could hold the bold kids or the useless kids or the mental kids or the thick kids in one room together. You know what people say, *Just get them all, put 'em on an island and let them do whatever they want to each other.* That was us. And, I suppose, when you think about it, that's Ireland.

So, our class was an Ireland within Ireland, a class full of misfits and weirdos. So much so that our teachers used to mitch off school. Like we didn't have to mitch, our teachers just regularly didn't come in. The number of sickies that were pulled on our class and, in fairness, why would they want to come in? What were they going to do if they did come in? Teach us what? Those of us that could learn had no interest or weren't able to sit down. And then the ones who were interested still couldn't spell their names. So, why would you bother?

In school I would perform at the back of the class and make everybody laugh, doing no work at all, but then I could go home and savage a book. The first book I ever got really into was *Animal Farm*. I loved it. I read it till it fell apart. And *Charlie and the Great Glass Elevator*, I was obsessed with it. There was a book called *Black Beach*, I think it was the first murder mystery novel I ever read, I couldn't stop or sleep, I was sunk into it. And all the Hardy Boys – I used to LOVE the Hardy Boys. There were a couple of lads at school who had them, so I'd get them through trades.

I knew I was good at stuff. I was funny, I could tell stories,

I took to language very well and song lyrics sit in my head forever. That was just a natural thing, but on its own it doesn't mean much, it's just a party trick. I wanted to write but I couldn't sit down long enough to concentrate. I couldn't study stuff and pass an exam. By the time I left school I'd come to believe that nothing that came easily to me had any value.

At one point I wanted to do archaeology because history was, by a long shot, the best subject they taught us. But, again, for that you needed maths and I was never going to get it. To make matters worse I could never hold down a job – everything I tried to earn a bit of cash as a teenager ended in disaster.

Selling programmes at Croke Park every Sunday seems straightforward enough, right? You'd get a little bib and you'd go out and sell your programmes. It was a penny for every programme you sold and a programme was a pound. So, you'd have to haul 300 of these yokes up Clonliffe Road on your back and sell them to boggers.

The problem was at the time there was this whole black market programme business going on. People were making their own programmes and flogging them. Ours were official but that didn't stop the boggers at every single game going, 'That's not the official programme.'

'It is the official programme, I'm wearing the bib!'

We got chased a lot by all the young lads because when you were wearing the bib but not carrying any programmes they knew you'd sold them all and your pockets were full of money. All the young lads from town hunted us down like prey, trying to get the three or four hundred quid in our pockets. You had to get that money back so you could get your £1.50 for your day's work. It was outrageous the cut.

One day I took off my bib when I was leaving but I didn't know what pile to put it on, so I just put it on any old pile. Some GAA fellow accused me of robbing the bib because obviously you could sell them for loads of money. If you were wearing the bib you could walk into Croke Park for free. That meant you could sell it to a guy who wanted to go to the All-Ireland for about 150 pounds. 'You sold it! You're not doing the programmes any more!' this guy shouted up the street at me. And that was the end of that.

There are so many examples of me messing or being disruptive in class. D'you remember when you were in school and dying to fart but knowing with absolute certainty it was going to be a whopper? Wondering, *How am I gonna do this?* The thing is once you fart in school you become Mr Shit-His-Pants for the rest of your life. Or for at least the next seven years.

So there I am. Dying to fart. Wondering how to save face. Solution: Do you remember those big heavy science textbooks? Well, I figured if I smashed one of them on the ground as hard as I could and farted at the same time I'd cover my tracks. That was the plan. So I lifted the book up over my head, smashed it on the ground and it went BANG! It was a massive sound, like a gunshot. The whole room went silent, everyone looking at me – like, *What did you do that for, you weirdo?* – and then I just farted really, really loudly.

Playing with gats was another big thing. Gats are makeshift catapults and this lad, Ronan, figured out how to make a gat by putting a pen in the ink holder and another pen in the hole in the desk and stretching a load of rubber bands between them. Then you folded up a load of paper into a kind of pellet and shot people with them.

One time I did the most amazing shot. It went round John M's head in a curve and shot him right up the hole; it looked like I shot him right in the sphincter. He screamed his head off because of the power of that shot; I swear to God it would've knocked a horse down.

Skinning people with rulers was another thing we did all the time. If someone skins you with a ruler it feels like they've cut a rasher off your hole. The pain of it.

The class I was in, we could really lose it sometimes and go feral. We had a teacher called Mr F and we broke the legs off the back of his chair and put the chair back on top, resting on them, so when he sat down, he went tumbling backwards into the wall.

Then there was a teacher called Mr C, who we thought was drunk all the time. We'd hide in the closet when he came in and make all these noises and he wouldn't know what was happening. Occasionally we'd throw our desks out the window. And poor Mrs D, she had a hard time with us. We'd let off bangers at the back of the class when Mrs D was in, scaring her almost half to death.

It was one thing after another. And I was always in the middle of it. Always in trouble. Shouting, roaring and making noise. It got to the point that a teacher would just walk in, point at me and say, 'Gallagher. Out. I'm not in the humour for you today.' At this stage, I didn't even wear a proper uniform any more. I was just a proper pain in the hole.

Outside of school things were going better for me. 1989 was the year when I first started to find my own bit of freedom and have new experiences like music and girls and kissing. At that time I was discovering punk music like Stiff Little Fingers, Dead Kennedys, Minor Threat. I was especially into

American punk, bands like 7 Seconds and The Descendents. At that age, mid-teens, music means so much to you, you never hear music again the way you hear it then. It's the same with people, you become cynical as you get older. It's very rare that you'll meet a new person and think:

'D'you know what? You're the best person ever, this is amazing, what d'you wanna do?'

'I don't know, what d'you fancy?'

'Let's just sit on a wall. Let's sit on a wall until everyone's worried sick about where we are and then we'll sit there a bit longer having the best fun ever.'

In 1989 I was fourteen and mad about girls, mad about them, but to ask a girl out I had to ring her and there was the strong likelihood one of her parents would answer the phone so I'd have to talk to them first. The whole thing was pure torture.

There was a phone under the stairs in our house, so if you were making a phone call everyone could hear you. The phone was a real 80s job, white with black buttons and a little volume dial at the bottom that didn't do anything no matter what you did.

Before anything else, before I even dialled the number, I had to make sure my parents weren't close by, earwigging. Then I had to make sure my sister wasn't around either. And then I had to have the guts to actually make the call, my sweaty little fourteen-year-old horny hands shivering. And then I'd ring, and her ma, or worse still, her da, would answer the phone.

'Hello, is Claire there?'

'Who's this?'

'Roger.' *(Oh no, why did I say that!)*

'Claire, there's a Roger on the phone!'

And then, 'Hello?'

'Hello, it's PJ.'

'My da said it was Roger.'

It was so embarrassing.

'I didn't want him to know it was me.'

'He doesn't know you.'

'I know . . . do you want to meet up with me or something?'

'No.'

'Okay then. Tell your da I said thanks.'

I wanted to swallow my own head with shame.

And then two weeks later, you fancy someone else, and you have to do it all over again.

'Hello.'

'Hello, who's that?'

'Roger.'

Oh God, why did I say that AGAIN?

'Roger who?'

'Eh . . . Roger Ramjet.'

'There's a Roger on the phone for you, Audrey. A Roger Ramjet on the phone.'

Oh my God, what is WRONG with me?

'Hello?'

'Yeah, it's PJ.'

'Why did you say it was Roger Ramjet?'

'I don't know, I always do that.'

'What do you mean you "always" do that?'

'I don't know. Do you want to meet up with me?'

'No.'

'Okay then.'

Brutal.

Another month goes by, you're back in the game . . .

'Hello?'

'Who's that?'

'Roger Ramjet.'

'Phyllis, there's a Roger Ramjet on the phone.'

'Hello?'

'It's PJ. Do you want to meet up with me?'

'Yeah.'

There's no way to describe the feeling without being corny. The best I can manage is that it's like listening to a power ballad and eating a bag of chips at the same time.

Phyllis was kind of my first big love. Full disclosure, that wasn't her real name, but she did have one of those old-fashionedy sounding names that stood out on a fourteen-year-old in the 80s. When she called over we went up into my bedroom. There were two single beds in my room and the walls and ceiling were covered with posters: AC/DC, Alice Cooper, Iron Maiden, The Misfits. Ted Nugent of all people – I don't think I really knew who he was at the time; he's turned into a crazy right-wing rocker. It was the best room I ever had; I wish I could get away with designing a room like that now.

I had my first kiss in that room with Phyllis. I hope it wasn't her first kiss because it would have put her off lads for life. We lay down on the bed and started giving each other frenchies. Frenchies was still a word – like, *did you get a frenchie off her?* What I didn't realize was that my tooth was leaning against her top lip and all my weight was on her and because we didn't know how to kiss it was just two wiggling tongues. One normal tongue and then mine.

I'm tongue-tied so it was just like a stump going in and around her mouth. She must have thought this was the most painful, horrible experience. I found out afterwards that my tooth was leaning on her top lip so much that she had to put a spoon in the freezer and put it on her lip to take the swelling down afterwards.

She was the first person I said 'I love you' to.

'I love you too. As a friend.'

Devastation.

Phyllis had had enough of me, and I was heartbroken. It's gas to think of it now but I was absolutely convinced my age was the problem. Her birthday is the 11th of April and mine is the 18th, so she was a week older than me. A week to the day. She was the first person I was close to who was also adopted. We had that in common and it meant a lot to me. Every year since 1989 I send her a happy birthday message on the 11th of April and whenever I bump into her I'm always delighted to see her and know she's doing well.

She had a friend Mary who is one of my oldest friends and is still a really good one. She was a big part of me recovering when I had my breakdown in 2021. Mary and I got together for a while when we were teenagers, soon after Phyllis and I broke up. We had to hide it because she was Phyllis's friend and friends weren't supposed to get with each other's exes. You know the way.

Mary came up with the idea of me following her to the Gaeltacht, so we could be together, but after two days in the Gaeltacht we broke up.

The Gaeltacht was in Donegal, everyone at it was a raging Provo. Everyone. It was a very lenient Irish college because the kids came from all over the north of Ireland and they weren't learning Irish at school. In fact one guy from Belfast was so good at Irish they made him speak French, that's how spiteful some people can be. Once again, going to show that effort never pays off!

When I got on the bus in Merrion Square my aul wan turned up and started crying all over me because I was going away for three weeks. I was like, 'Jesus Christ, why are you embarrassing me like this? I'm fourteen years old. Get over yourself!'

Two things I remember from that day: my ma crying on me before I got on the bus; and a British soldier in khaki camouflage gear and brandishing an assault rifle, getting on the bus and walking up and down checking us all out. My ma crying was way more horrific than that.

That trip was my first taste of being properly away from the family, away from that house, meeting people in a different environment, hanging out with people my own age. It was just deadly.

12.

Matchstick mickey shit sticks

Am I working-class? I don't really know. There was never any money. When my ma was on the dole she never let on. 'I have to go to my office and collect my wages,' and off we'd go into town. It wasn't till I was on the dole myself and I went into the dole office on Seán McDermott Street and thought, 'Oh, this used to be my ma's office,' that the penny dropped.

Clontarf was posh but we totally stuck out there – a gaff with a family of misfits and six loonies. And I never aspired to finish school or go to college or any of that.

So, you tell me, I don't know.

If I could wave a wand and have the successful career of my dreams it would be motor racing; that's what I would've loved to have done professionally. Growing up all I wanted to do was play football for the Dubs, but the only way I can catch a ball is with my face. When I was in school I wanted to write but I couldn't sit down long enough to concentrate.

But the one thing I can do is stand up and tell a story. There is a weird reality check in that, because I was always looking at my old man and thinking, 'Okay. Get real. You can't do what you want to do, you have to do what you're good at, so just get on with it.' And then I found myself, years later, in the same boat he was.

This is a fellow who never really expressed himself, just came and went all the time, tried to avoid awkward situations. Much like myself. I would stay up all night if it meant I could avoid a conversation during the day, and that pretty much was the same with him. He wasn't a communicator, not at all. My ma was the communicator. My ma never stopped communicating. My ma over-communicated. I'm a mixture of the two of them because I'll do anything to avoid communicating with you, but when I have to, I can do it very well.

There's absolutely nothing I wouldn't do to not be at parties, not be at weddings, not be in friends' houses, not be in any social situations. Yet, because I know how to express myself, for years I made a living by being in a room with lots of people. Doing stand-up was a form of torture because every single night I'd know – not think, I'd *know* – 'This is going to be the worst night ever, this is the night where everybody realizes I'm absolutely useless.'

But it never happened. Even the bad nights ended up being great stories for the following night. Unquestionably, I have some knack for communication.

The problem is I've always been good at stuff I don't rate and never any good at the things I actually want to be good at. You know all this, 'You can do anything you want'? You can't. You have to be good at it first. And if you don't want to do what you're good at – tough, you're stuck with it.

That's how it is for me with stand-up. People will say it's a great art form. It's a great art form when you're talking to the taxman all right. Outside of that, stand-up is scribbling, the verbal equivalent of graffiti. If even. And I don't mean graffiti as in Maser or Spice Bag; I mean matchstick mickeys on the back of the toilet door.

'I rode your ma in this toilet.'

'For sex, call Jimmy on 087 . . . ', whatever.

Stand-ups aren't artists. Not at all. But am I an artist for the purpose of this book and the tax exemption? Absolutely. My artist exemption certificate is in my house framed on the wall.

At school I always wanted to play Gaelic but I couldn't catch a ball. Then I tried out for rugby but had the same problem. I'd be out on the pitch breaking me balls, but I couldn't get picked for any games, even a friendly. Just couldn't catch a ball.

Then a rugby coach took me to one side, and he goes, 'You're looking at the game all wrong. You're jumping to try and catch things. Instead, watch the way the ball goes and hit the guy that gets it. Forget trying to get the ball. You've no coordination. The ball's no good to you. Don't even try to stop other people getting it. Wait till they catch it, wait till they're holding it, and hit them. You just make sure they can't move when they get it. Just hit them.'

And he goes, 'Run into people as hard as you can. You're great at hitting people. You're fearless out there.'

That changed everything. In no time I'm getting picked for all the games, getting brought on all the away trips. Now, I'm going out to the southside beating teams that are really good. There's this big, positive change – all because I've found a new way of looking at something.

It would have been hard to drown out all the negativity I was getting from everywhere else, including inside my own head, so this intervention had a big impact on me. It was one of the best moments of my school days. I saw an alternate way of looking at a problem that seemed impossible.

More to the point, someone saw something in me. This brilliant man took a minute out of his day to take a kid aside and say, 'I give a shit, and here's what you're gonna do.' To have that encouragement, to hear that you're able to do something that's not disruptive in life. Just to hear someone go, 'Good man,' for the first time ever. That stayed with me for a long time.

From early on we all knew that nobody would be worrying about how many points I got in the Leaving Cert. Least of all me. The only question was: how would the torture end? Naturally, I went for a big bang exit. It's the only way to make a clean break of anything. The whole thing came to a head over an accidental case of dreadlocks.

Most kids can do what they want with their hair – they get into metal and they grow their hair long. They get into The Cure and they grow their hair wide. They get into punk and they grow a mohawk. What I have on my head, though, is an uncontrollable force. One time I tried to grow my hair long and I grew a beard on the back of my head. It wasn't a successful look. Bum fluff on my face and a full beard on the back of my head.

So, that had to go. After that I tried to grow a rockabilly-style fringe. I thought 'I'll grow this fringe and shave the rest of my hair off and that'll be kind of punk.' But it wasn't, because I've curly hair. After that, when I was sixteen I went for this hairstyle, if you could actually call it a 'style', that the lads I was in school with liked to call 'the shit sticks'. I had five big thick dreadlocks hanging down the front of my face.

Literally. They went from my forehead to underneath my chin, covering my acne basically. Kids used to call me the Bermuda Triangle because it was like a face went in there one day and never came out.

Problem is you can't see when you've five heavy dread-locks covering your face. So, I'd tuck them behind my ear. After a while they curled around my ear naturally from being there all the time. It looked like this filthy hairy dead animal was hanging off the centre of my head and had sort of wrapped itself down one side of my face and tried to walk its way back up again. It was only a matter of time before this disgusting, stupid, ugly *thing* on my head got me into trouble. Because nobody would walk around like that. Nobody.

At this point I've done my Inter Cert but I haven't gone on to fourth year. Instead, I'm doing this thing called VPTP – vocational preparation and training programme. All the misfits were put into the VPTP. Academically, we did not progress past third year.

We're only back in school a few weeks, not even a month, and one of the teachers tells me to cut my hair. I was like, right, here we go. I've just spent the whole summer growing shit sticks and, grand, they look ridiculous, but they're my shit sticks. So I went home, and I cut them myself to the end of my nose, and I went in the next day and he goes, 'No, you're gonna cut them properly off, you look like a gouger.' I think it was 'gouger'. I can't remember the exact word he said but it was one of those words only a teacher in the 90s would get away with. And that was it. I had reached my limit with school; I couldn't handle it any more.

So, I told him to fuck off. And then I went round all of the teachers going, 'You can fuck off and you can fuck off and you can fuck off and you can fuck off.' Then I went up to the form master's office but he wasn't there so I waited. When he sees me he goes, 'What are you doing here?' He had this ridiculous quacky ducky voice. And I said, 'You see, you? You can fuck off.'

And then I went looking for Mr D, one of the cool teachers. Mr Kool. One of the kids said to him once, 'You have a lot of stories, don't you? Pity none of them ever happened.' That kid got into the biggest amount of trouble ever. It was hilarious because it was spot-on.

I told Mr D, 'I'm leaving and I'm never coming back.' And he said, 'Well, we'll see what your parents have to say about that.' Little did he know my parents.

My ma was relieved that I was leaving school. Her only concern was that she didn't want me idle. 'Whatever you do, you're not sitting around this house all day.' To be fair, she already had six patients and me aul fella sitting around the house. Last thing she needed was another fella under her feet.

The problem was, I didn't really know what to do. All I was interested in was doing something in music. I liked music and I was playing in bands – now, the worst bands in the world, although we thought they were great.

Everyone was in a band then. You had to be in a band, otherwise what were you doing with your time? Everyone wanted to play guitar or be a singer, but if you were a bass player or a drummer, you could take a pick of the bands because nobody wanted to be a bass player or a drummer. So, I was like, okay then, I'll be a bass player. Apart from the gap in the market for bass players, it seemed easier than guitar – there's four strings on the bass and six strings on the guitar so I reckoned it would be four times easier to play. That's how good I am at maths.

The first band I was in was called Bored Stiff. We were more band by committee though, because we had no instruments. Then when we finally got some instruments, we didn't know how to tune them and the lad who'd been saying he could sing for the past two years went suddenly mute.

'I can't sing in front of youse!'

'Well then, how are you gonna sing in front of thousands of people?' Couldn't even tune our guitars and worried about audiences of thousands.

Eventually I got into a proper band, a punk band called Black Rain. We did a gig in the attic of the White Horse Inn on George's Quay in town. We were all sixteen, so technically we weren't allowed into the pubs and some of our friends couldn't get in without fake IDs. At the time you had to pay twenty-five quid for the stage, and we made and printed our own tickets and posters. People came into town to see us, and it was kind of successful.

Your man running it wanted us to finish at half ten but we were having such a good time we just kept playing, so he jumped on to the stage and turned off all the electricity and threw us out. It was great. The whole night was a savage buzz. The kudos of being in a band, being able to tell people you were in a band that actually had instruments and actually played music.

We were probably brutal though. We must have been brutal because here I am all these years later and I can't play bass. But we did it, we pulled it off. The strongest memory I have from that night was standing at the bar and ordering a pint of Guinness. I was so happy I got served a pint of Guinness but when I went to pick it up, I pushed it off the counter and it landed in a woman's handbag.

Nothing spilled. Not a drop. Not one drop anywhere. It

just disappeared into the handbag. So, I just bought another one.

My folks bought the bass guitar for me in Musicmaker on Exchequer Street – a hundred and eighteen quid I think it was back in the day. They bought me an amp too, but it didn't last long because one of my mates, his da threw it at his head and smashed it all up. That lad is a conspiracy theorist now.

I've never liked being in big bustling rooms. I didn't go to nightclubs. Lads going out to clubs trying to get their hole? Nah. No *Tomango's Where the Gang Goes* for me. None of that. When all that E and raves came on to the scene, I hated the thought of it. Sitting in the corner of a pub wanting to have a laugh, that was always my thing. Music gigs were okay because they were controlled – back then you'd watch the band for an hour and then hang out together and have a chat.

Even saying that, though, I had no real interest in going to gigs unless I was doing the gig. Being passive didn't interest me at all. Whenever I went into a venue, I knew exactly which side of the stage I wanted to be on. That's something that's never changed. There's nothing on this earth that would get me in to watch a stand-up show. It's the same with radio, people always ask what radio I listen to. Radio? I do in me hole listen to the radio. The only time I listen to the radio is when I'm doing it myself.

People always say you need to be influenced by the best. If you want to be a good actor, you've got to go to loads of plays. If you want to be a stand-up, you have to go see loads of stand-ups.

If you want to be like every other arsehole out there, that's good advice. There's a reason when you go to comedy and listen to the radio that everything sounds the exact same. It's because they're all listening to each other. So, if you want to formulate rules in your head and you want to be told this is the way to do things or this is how things are done, well, by all means go and knock any originality you have out of yourself.

My advice is the exact opposite: *Watch nothing. Do whatever you want. There are no rules.* Really pay attention to what you are doing and nobody else. That's always been my philosophy anyway.

So I was still playing in the bands and thinking that that was the main thing that I wanted. But see, that's the thing, I was never aiming for success in any of this. I just wanted to kind of be good at it. None of us were thinking, 'Oh we're gonna tour the world.' It was only, 'Maybe we'll get to do gigs and have fun and make a couple of quid.'

It was about being different as well. Standing out. Looking for a way to survive when you couldn't survive in the real world. No maths, no discipline, and I couldn't do the same thing every day. As far as I knew I was going to be unemployed for the rest of my life. Might as well learn an instrument and have some fun.

Wanting to be different, if I was to analyse it, was most likely about needing attention. The desperate insecurity of being adopted, not knowing the situation and thinking that you were given away because you weren't wanted. Trying to get attention at home and never being able to do it. Asking people to stop drinking and never having any success. Being a disruptive nuisance at school. Positive attention is what I was after, and that's something an audience can give you.

That need is why you end up walking on stage expecting a round of applause. You're asking strangers to like you all the time, and the only way to get strangers to like you all the time is to be different or at least provoke some reaction out of them.

To escape the feeling of being ignored you have to be different, walking around with shit sticks hanging out of your head, wearing tartan trousers and Doc Martens up to your knees, and playing bass guitar because everybody else was playing the guitar.

13.

Best use of a human head

My ma was always a very enterprising woman, so soon as I told her I wanted to do something with music she found out about the Sound Training Centre and asked me if I'd be willing to go for training there.

'If I can get into it, I'll do it. A hundred per cent.'

As much as she didn't want me hanging around the house, it's not exactly where I wanted to be either.

When I started I was only sixteen and so much younger than everyone else in there. There were people there in their thirties, and even the ones in their mid-twenties seemed very old to me. Weirdly enough, the only other sixteen-year-old on the course was my cousin; the two of us were just kids.

Everyone at the Sound Training Centre wanted to be sound engineers. They wanted to work in the studios, or they wanted to be behind the sound desk at big gigs. I decided to study lighting because lighting was different. My reasoning: if everyone's doing sound then it'll probably be easier to get a job in lighting.

The Sound Training Centre was where my friend Luca's restaurant Rosa Madre is now on Crow Street in Temple Bar. Temple Bar was a hole back then; the whole area was run down to hell. But it was deadly being there. Rents were cheap and there were loads of scrappy little businesses run out of semi-derelict buildings. Second-hand shops. People doing artsy stuff. Such a different world, an opening to a cool world. Doing that course was the beginning of a new way of seeing the world and the start of finally being able to get behind something.

It was only four months of training. Four months and it cost 1,600 quid. It was wild money at the time. I applied for a student card so I could get discounts and stuff. The USIT people who issued the cards to college students were debating whether to give it to me or not because I was only going to be there for four months. I got one in the end.

In lighting they gave you the basics of how to design a light show so you could try and go and get work. It was less 'Here's how you do it' and more 'Here's the bare bone basics – now go out and hustle a bit.' They taught you how to plug guitars into amps, the rough basics of how a lighting desk worked and some sound engineering, how to operate a sound desk and work in a recording studio. There was a test at the end, and you needed 40 per cent to pass, but because I couldn't figure out any of the recording studio stuff (numbers again) I only got 35 per cent.

Before I left, one of the tutors had asked a load of us to go to a training session where he was being assessed as a teacher. I went but most people didn't. Afterwards he said, what do you want? We can give you some extra marks for turning up. I said, 'Gimme five per cent.' That's how I passed and got my certificate.

Not long after that I went up to Lighting Dimensions, this big warehouse that was opposite the Meath Hospital on Long Lane in Dublin 8. I walked in the door and asked for some work experience and a few days later I was sweeping the floor.

I'll never forget my first pay cheque: 32 pounds and 32 pence. Unbelievable. I really felt I'd arrived. Finally, made something out of my life. *This is it. I have a job.* When I left the band it caused a lot of trouble but there was no money in it. It was going to take a very long time for me to make 32 pounds and 32 pence playing bass guitar in a punk band.

I was really into BMXs at the time so I cycled a BMX from Clontarf into Long Lane every day. A BMX! I couldn't even sit down on the thing. But I loved going into work every day. There was a guy called Jason Byrne who worked at a desk fixing and making lamps. Jason, it turned out, was both hilarious and going to change the course of my life. If this was having a job, I loved it. Every day was unbelievable craic.

Lighting Dimensions was owned by a company called White Light in England and they sent over this new manager one time to try and turn the company around. We tied him up, put him in a flight case and called a courier, who delivered him to the Olympia Theatre. Can you imagine doing that now? No. Can you imagine putting a human being in a box, tied up, and having them delivered to another place? And not being fired or arrested?

The courier came back with the manager sitting in the passenger seat and we all thought it was the funniest thing.

When you started there you got tied to a lamppost or gaffer-taped up and thrown into the skip for a couple of hours. So, when I started there they got me out on the street, gaffer-taped me on to a lamppost, put a birdcage over my head and left me at the side of the road. The guards pulled up, got out of the car and asked me what was going on. I said, 'I work in there,' nodding over at the warehouse where all these heads were sticking out of the door watching us. The guards laughed their heads off, got into the car and drove off.

I really loved that place. It was so chaotic. We used to electrocute each other all the time for fun, put bare wires into a toolbox and when someone went rooting around for a tool whack the plug in and electrocute them.

There was a carpet guy around the back and occasionally we would roll people up in a carpet. I'll tell you something, if you're rolled up in 300 metres of carpet, you're not getting out. You'll be stuck in there for the day.

The only time I ever got upset about being tied up was when they were cutting me out of some gaffer tape and the Stanley blade cut through my skin by accident. But that was the only time.

One day instead of building lights for Van Morrison or whoever we were supposed to be building lights for, we decided we were going to have a Wild West Day instead. We made cowboy hats out of the light fittings and played country music all day long.

Nobody did much work, but we did enough to get by. The place functioned, just about – but it was mental. One time Jason got a letter from his girlfriend excusing him from work. His girlfriend!

Mostly all we did was listen to music all day and hang mirror balls from the ceiling. For Jason's birthday one year we put some scaffold across the roof with two motors on it. We tied him to it with a mirror ball hanging out of his chest and left him rotating up on the roof for the day.

One time I broke my shoulder doing bike tricks, going down to the jumps and the chuckies at St Anne's Park on my BMX. I took a month off work. A month! Nobody said a word. Occasionally I would cycle in and hang out there because I missed the place, but I didn't do any work. It was a great time. It was everything the VTPT should have been but wasn't. You were never going to leave Lighting Dimensions and get a regular job.

The English people running the place just couldn't believe the carry-on. They sent another manager over, again to try and straighten us out. Her nickname was Cheese Roll because every day she'd go to Spar for a cheese roll. It was the beginning of all that, the birth of the Spar Deli. She did her best to try and straighten us out, but of course the place closed down. It had to close down. It could never have continued in that vein.

Jason was always ambitious, more ambitious than anyone else I'd ever met, to be honest. He was the ambitious one who had the idea of leaving Lighting Dimensions to go to work for a new company that was setting up called Arena Lighting. He said I should go with him. We were doing comedy stuff together – a bit of stand-up in pubs in town – he said he was going to keep doing it. And if that didn't work out, we'd have this job to fall back on.

When Jason started doing comedy he didn't want to do it on his own, he wanted someone to come with him, so we'd write these sketches together. Jason would get up and he would do about ten minutes of stand-up and then he'd do this thing where he'd say, 'Are there any volunteers in the audience for my next bit?' I would always volunteer.

It would start with him saying, 'So, have we ever met

before?' and me saying no. That was pretty much the only thing I'd ever say, and then we'd act out these sketches where my body would be used as a prop and I made funny faces.

The sketches we were doing at the time were in the International and the Norseman and the White Horse, real small clubs. I wasn't telling jokes. I was a human prop, a stooge – the kick-in-the-arse lad. But still, there was an audience and it was something different.

That was when I won my first award, 'Best use of a human head' at the Comedy Cellar. Amazingly, I was the only person in the category, nobody else was nominated. I was really chuffed, and I got this plaque with some kind of Asian-looking writing on it that I kept for years and years.

Then years later I won a Comedy Gent and I think that was the last year the awards happened. Comedy Gent sounds like something you'd get in trouble for now, but Deirdre O'Kane won it one year so it wasn't just for gents.

The award I missed out on was the Simon Fiver. Simon was a guy that worked in the International Comedy Club from the very start, and every year he would choose who got a fiver from him. It became a prestigious thing because Simon saw every single show, no one else did. I never won the Simon Fiver. Fuck you, Simon.

14.

The young Fenian

At Arena Lighting we weren't just servicing parts to send out to gigs. We were making everything from scratch, putting all the parts together and sending it all out to venues. Jason made the lights; I made all the cables. It was very hard work at the start.

It was while working in Arena Lighting that I had my first proper mental breakdown, when I was twenty-two. A load of us had been over in Halifax for the weekend, for a bit of craic. Soon after we came back, I was watching Oprah Winfrey and I saw a man having a heart attack in the audience. Watching him have a heart attack I thought I was having a heart attack too.

Convinced I was dying, I went downstairs to my ma and she gave me a bottle of Guinness. She thought I had the fear, so she was giving me a cure to get me back on the straight and narrow. But I didn't have the fear, I was fucked up. Like really, really fucked up.

I didn't leave the house for months and months, couldn't leave the house, couldn't function, couldn't think, couldn't lie down, couldn't distract myself, nothing. All these really horrible, weird images of dead bodies in my head and crazy religious polluted stuff. I was literally tormented, in total despair.

When these horrible thoughts are bombarding you, it's hard not to think that you must be a horrible person. Otherwise, why would they be in your head? You don't understand that you're so disturbed by these thoughts because you *don't* like them; you think you're having these thoughts because you *do*. The more I tried to block them the worse they got and I was trapped in a vicious cycle – frightening thoughts going round and round and round until I was completely incapacitated.

A doctor told me to put my runners on and get some exercise. I tried to tell him, 'There's something wrong here, this isn't normal, this feeling, whatever it is, it's not normal.' He said, 'I'm not going to even entertain that. I'm not going to even entertain that nonsense for one minute.'

He was telling me I was okay, and I was telling him I was not. He had absolutely put me down as a chancer.

Finally, my ma said, 'We have to get you a psychiatrist.' I was afraid to go, afraid of the medication. Afraid I'd take one tablet and be staring at a wall for the next thirty years in a straitjacket in a padded cell. So I was holding off, thinking, *Maybe I'll get better. Maybe I will. Maybe.*

And then I got to the point where I knew, I just knew, I was never going to get better. I was never getting out of the place I was in. And, *Why not?* You resign yourself. *Why not?*

She wanted me to go and see this guy she'd seen on TV, Anthony Clare. He turned out to be the best man ever. Just this great psychiatrist, straight up. He asked me to tell him what was going on and I said, 'I don't think I can.'

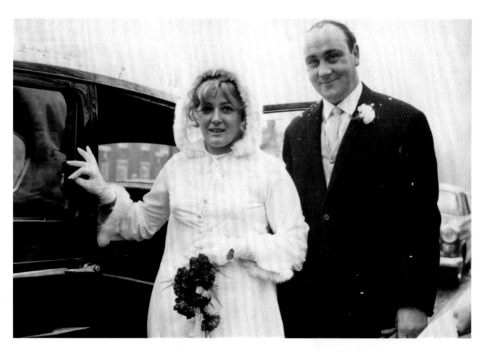

Meet the parents: Helen and Sean's wedding in January 1969.

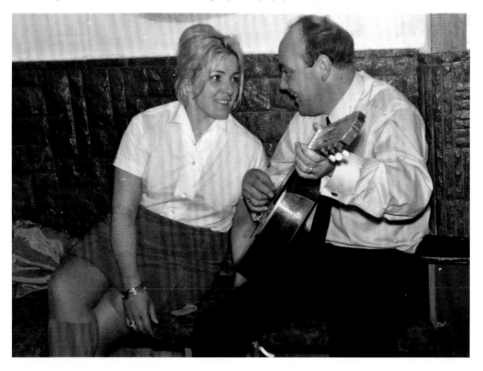

Sean serenading Helen on their honeymoon in Torremolinos.

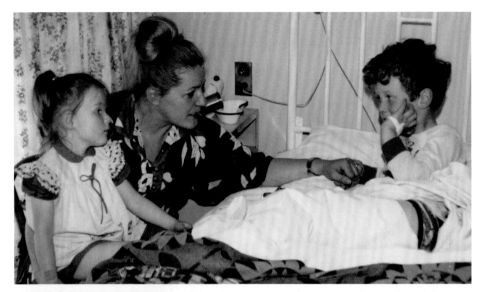

(*Above*) Ma and Stacey visiting me in hospital. I'm about five, getting my adenoids out.

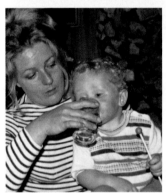

(*Left*) With Ma in early 1976. The xylophone mallet was probably going to end up behind the dog's ear – Tara was a saint.

(*Below left*) Looking mystified by the grown-ups celebrating my birthday – it was any excuse for a party in our house.

(*Below right*) Stacey just turned up one day out of the blue when I was nearly three.

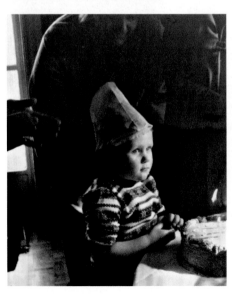

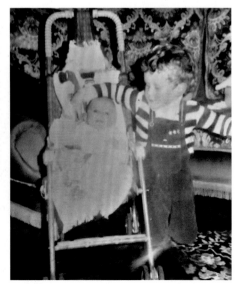

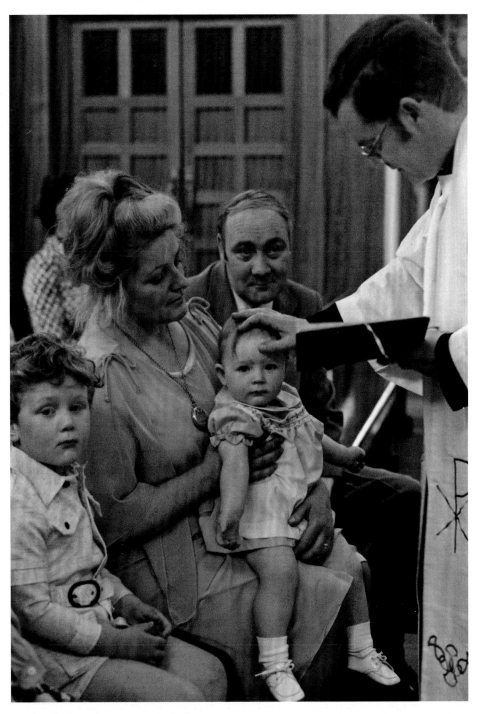

Stacey and I were christened together in a two-for-one deal. I wasn't too impressed by the event, but the promise of McDonald's afterwards made it an easier sell.

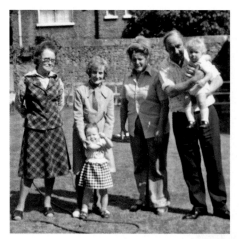

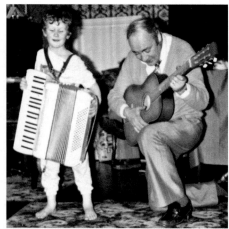

(*Above*) With my parents and two grannies, Gallagher (*left*) and Kirwan. The other child is my cousin Ailish. We always called Granny Gallagher 'Ma'am' and this picture was taken in her back garden.

(*Top right*) Da and me in Ma'am's house.

(*Right*) Got up like a dandy for my First Communion when all the other fellas looked like extras from *Miami Vice*.

(*Below*) On our big 1984 American trip we visited Ma's younger sister, Stacey (*left*, with Ma), and her family in Arizona. In the foreground is our Egyptian lodger, Zsu Zsu, who came with us.

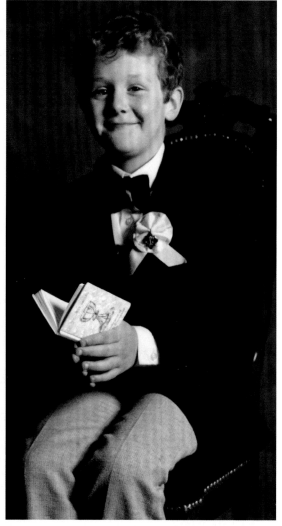

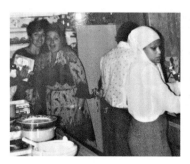

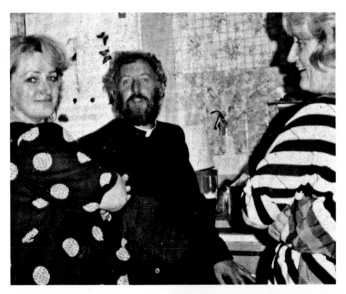

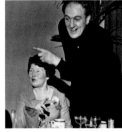

The infamous Fr Michael Cleary at Ma and Da's wedding reception. (The Wolfe Tones were the wedding band. The woman is probably our grandaunt Bid, Granny Gallagher's sister.)

(*Above*) Ma (*left*) loved a bit of religion. Pictured with her sister Anne and their friend, and scourge of the devil, Fr Mick Maher.

(*Right*) Rocking my George Best underpants, with my American cousin Dakota Clark in 1984.

(*Below left*) Hanging out with the community garda, Seán O'Neill, in Fairview. Garda O'Neill cycled around on an old-fashioned bike and dropped in often. He enjoyed a drink with my parents.

(*Below right*) Growing up all I wanted to do was play football for the Dubs, but the only way I can catch a ball is with my face.

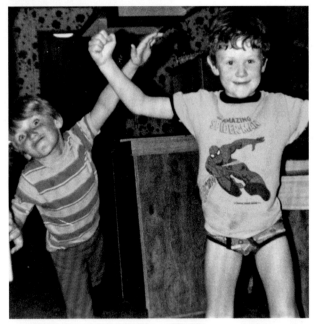

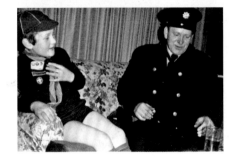

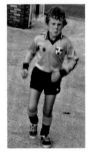

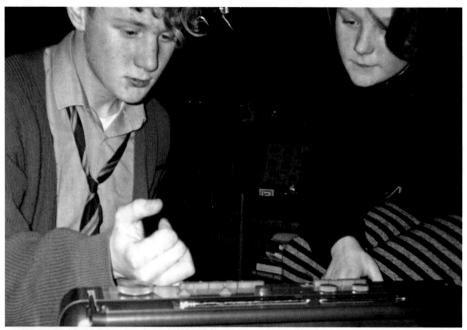

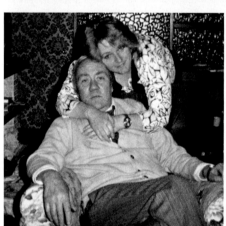

(*Above*) Stacey and me with our first ghetto blaster. Our ma forced us to pose, saying she wanted 'a picture of you two getting on'.

(*Left*) Sean and Helen in our house in Clontarf, around the late 1980s.

(*Below left*) My attempt to grow a rockabilly-style fringe. The 'style' mutated into dreadlocks. They got me kicked out of school.

(*Below*) Gurning with my friend 'A' (Aidan) AKA 'Face'. He was called Face for obvious reasons – the face is still a thing of beauty.

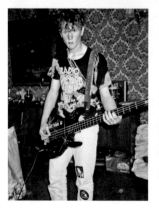

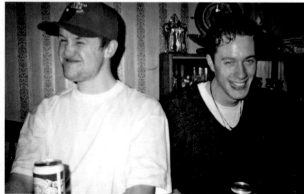

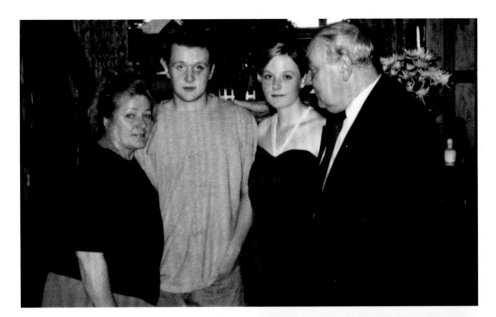

(*Above*) Stacey in the traditional pre-Debs family photo in the mid-90s. My black eye is kind of a downer though.

(*Right*) With Stacey at her eighteenth birthday party.

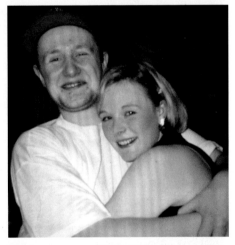

(*Below left*) I met Jason Byrne at my first job. Jason was hilarious and would change the course of my life.

(*Below right*) More posing as a happy family: my twenty-first and Da is presenting me with the symbolic key of the door.

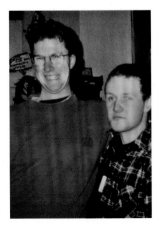

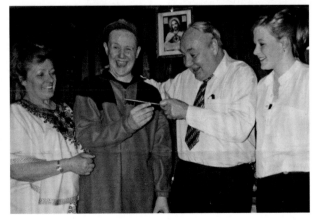

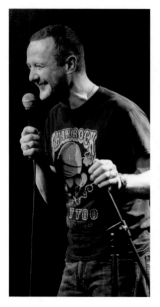

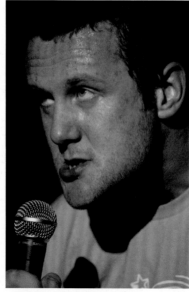

(*Left*) I might not have been the best joke writer, but nobody worked harder doing stand-up than I did.

(*Right*) I ended up in this state after every performance, just relieved to have survived. The pressure of delivering a good show felt like a massive weight on my shoulders.

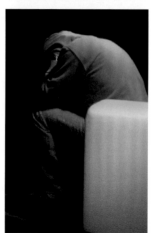

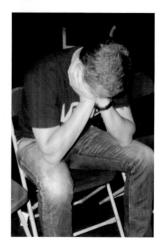

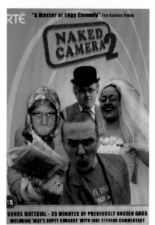

(*Far left*) People still remember Jake Stevens from *Naked Camera*. He's the kind of obnoxious know-all we've all met.

(*Left*) Jake and the Dirty Aul Wan on a *Naked Camera* DVD cover. Maeve Higgins as the Desperate Bride and Patrick McDonnell as Clifford the Orangeman.

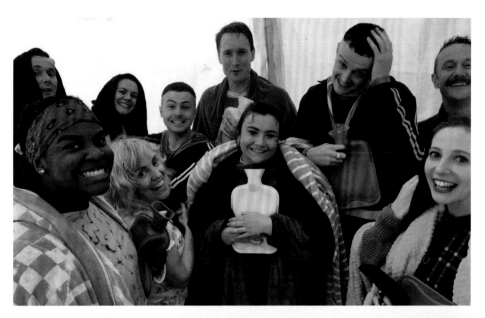

(*Above*) With *The Young Offenders* cast at the end of shooting the third season, which went out in 2020. We thought it would be the last season, but season four is out in 2024.

(*Right*) On *The Young Offenders* set as school principal Barry Walsh. Considering how much I hated school, playing Barry is the height of irony.

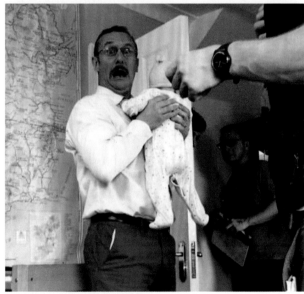

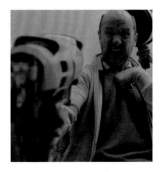

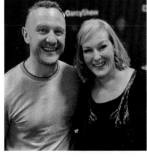

(*Far left*) Playing Ray the drug dealer in *The Young Offenders* movie. I threw myself into that audition.

(*Left*) Promoting the play *Madhouse* with Katherine Lynch. *Madhouse* is based on my early years and Katherine played my ma.

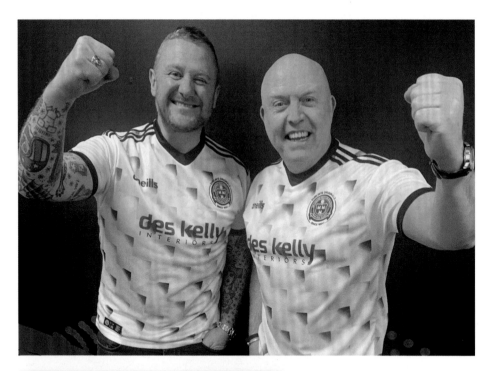

(*Above*) This picture has everything – with Jim McCabe, my great pal and Radio Nova breakfast show co-host, showing off the 2023 Bohs away strip. Bohs is the best team ever. Presenting radio is the best job ever.

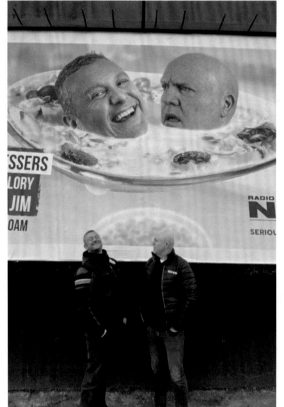

(*Left*) Jim and me admiring Nova's new billboard advertising *Morning Glory with PJ and Jim*. They call us 'cereal messers' – they're not wrong.

(*Below*) In my happy place: behind the mic in Nova. I love this job.

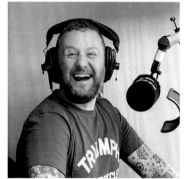

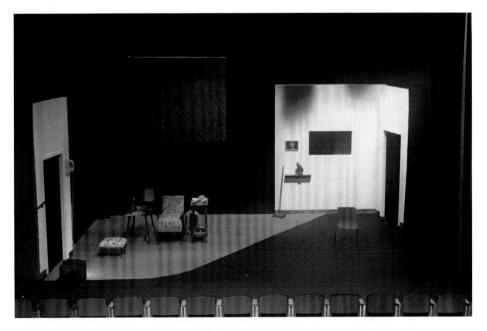

The *Madhouse* set during the 2019 tour, snapped on my phone before the show. The play was a comic telling of my childhood featuring Katherine Lynch as Ma, her armchair front and centre. The set is deceptively peaceful-looking considering the mayhem that would kick off once the curtain went up.

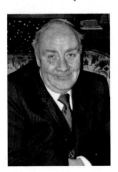

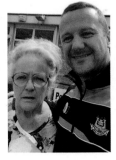

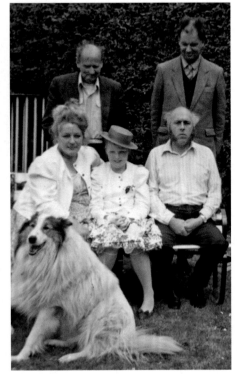

(*Above left*) Da was fifty-eight when he died and this picture is from years earlier. Time took a big toll on him.

(*Above right*) Ma and me after voting in the 2015 marriage equality referendum. She wasn't far off ninety when she died in November 2022 – which was impressive considering the life she'd had.

(*Right*) Ma with Stacey on her Confirmation Day, along with three of our lodgers: Little Joe, Big Joe and Danny. Skippy the dog had a brain tumour, so also had his issues.

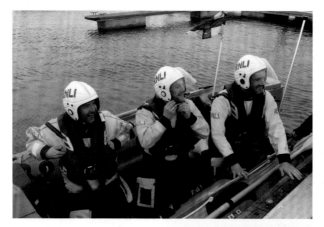

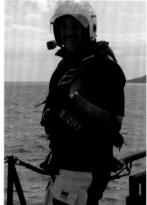

(*Above*) Volunteering has been a big part of my life. It's not that I'm a great fellow; I get more out of it than I give. Here I am (*centre*) on an RNLI dinghy.

(*Above right*) On an RNLI call-out. It was a good day; nobody died.

(*Right*) Blood Bikes is an amazing outfit, transporting urgent medical samples and supplies.

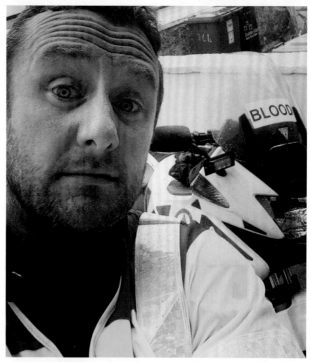

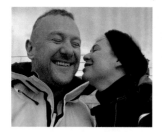

(*Above*) With Kelly at the 2022 Christmas Eve RNLI lifeboat memorial in Dún Laoghaire.

(*Right*) Bundled up for RNLI duties, wearing a Bohs hat.

(*Far right*) A face (*far right*) in the crowd in Tolka Park. Bohs had just scored against Shelbourne!

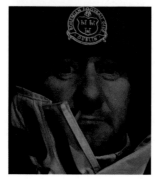

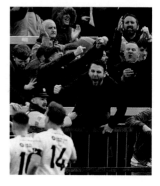

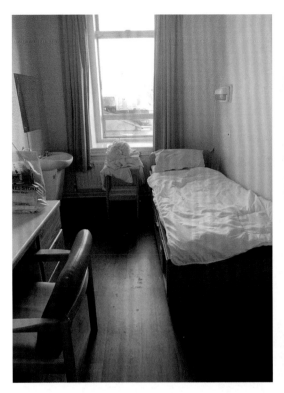

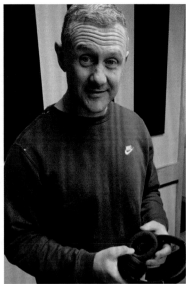

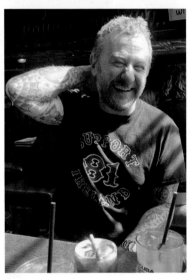

(*Above*) My room in St Patrick's Hospital. It could have been a suite in the Shelbourne I was so glad to be there.

(*Above right*) Before. The last picture taken of me, at work in October 2021, before I went into St Pat's. I was in bits inside.

(*Right*) After. Celebrating my forty-eighth birthday in April 2023.

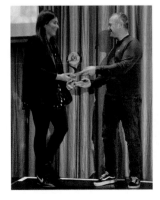

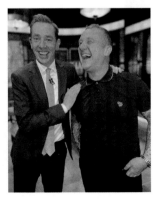

(*Far left*) Presenting my best friend Stefanie Preissner with an award at the 2022 Mental Health Media Awards.

(*Left*) I got a huge reaction to discussing my breakdown with Ryan Tubridy on *The Late Late Show* in October 2022. Ryan was in touch again long afterwards, making sure I was doing okay.

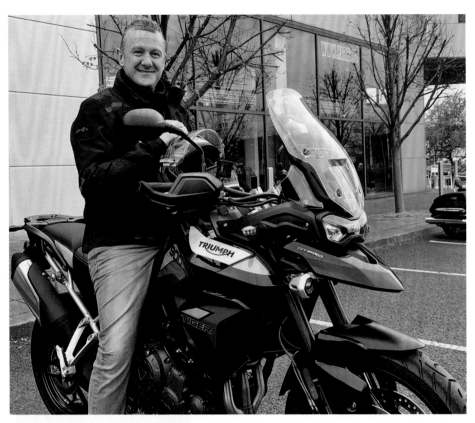

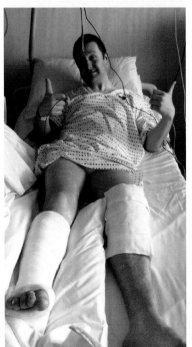

(*Above*) I went a bit mad buying bikes when I got out of Pats. This is my Triumph Tiger. I bought a Harley too.

(*Left*) April 2011, after one of my many motorbike-racing accidents. Racing was worth every injury and I regret nothing.

(*Below*) In Mondello, 2008. The rush of racing feeds your soul. It is the best sport ever.

(*Below right*) Hanging out with bikers is one of life's great pleasures. With mates Shane Bradley (*left*) and Matt 'Bratt' Kelly, an actual Hells Angel.

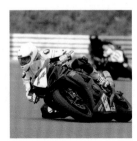

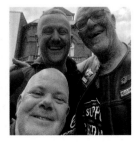

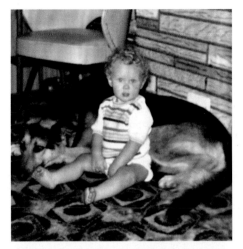

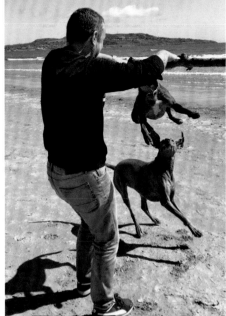

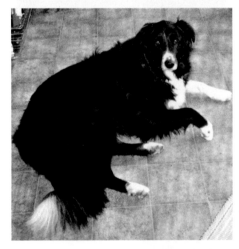

(*Top left*) Tara was my first pal in life. Dogs have been my best friends since I was a baby.

(*Left*) Our last family dog, Saoirse – the greatest animal ever.

(*Above*) With Stella, the Staffy (*top*), and Wendy, the Weimaraner. I share them with my ex-wife, Elaine.

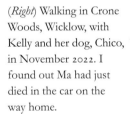

(*Right*) Walking in Crone Woods, Wicklow, with Kelly and her dog, Chico, in November 2022. I found out Ma had just died in the car on the way home.

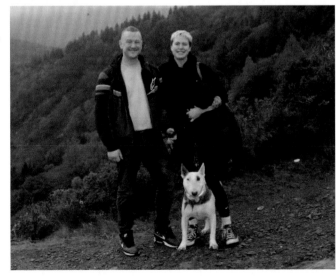

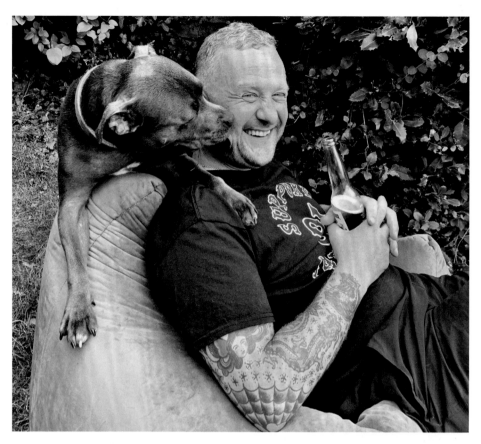

Hanging out with Stella. She has an anxiety disorder, but she's coming around. We're both getting better by the day.

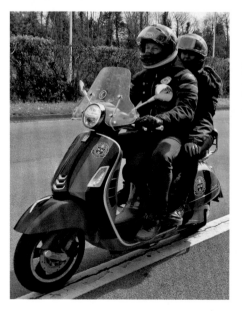

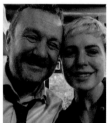

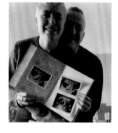

(*Left*) If this included a dog it would be my life in one shot: on a bike, in Bohs colours, Kelly on the back, the twins already on board.

(*Above left*) Kelly and I met marching under the Bohs banner at the 2022 Dublin Pride Parade.

(*Above right*) Our first sighting of Stevie and Milo. Being handed that scan was when we found out we were having twins.

'Well, what are you doing here then? If you don't tell me I can't do anything for you.'

So I spit out everything. Told him about the horrible thoughts and images. And he was really reassuring. Dr Clare said the main thing I had to understand was that these thoughts disturbed me and that was what was causing me the problem. He said if I was a bad person, I'd be indulging these thoughts, wanting to go out and enact them. But instead, I hated them, they were intrusive and not at all enjoyable. He put me on antidepressant medication and told me it would take a few weeks to kick in.

Within two weeks I do remember feeling that I was coming back to myself. The first night I was able to go out and handle a crowd and live my life again, I went to see James Brown in the Point Depot. For the first time in a long time, I had a bit of hope. But I'd lost my job, I was unemployed, the whole lot. My mates weren't gone, but my job was.

Truth is I'd never really liked the whole night-time work and overnight shifts at Arena Lighting; I had preferred the regularity of being in the warehouse at Lighting Dimensions.

What I'd *really* enjoyed doing were the sketches with Jason, but Jason was moving on in the comedy world, doing more stand-up, so the sketch shows were starting to die off. I was really at a loose end, like a proper loose end. And that's when I joined Sinn Féin.

Republicanism was always a big thing in our house; my ma was a mad Fenian. My dad on the other hand had no nationalist leanings, but he'd say he had because he'd always tell you whatever it was you wanted to hear. If you were a Unionist and you told my da what you thought, and asked, 'What do you think about that?' he'd agree with you completely on everything. A hundred per cent. 'Couldn't agree more, *God Save the Queen*, would you like a pint?'

If you were a member of the IRA hiding a grenade in a sandwich and said, 'Would you look after that grenade for me, Sean?' he'd say, 'Come on Ireland, *Tiocfaidh ár lá*. Absolutely. A hundred per cent. D'you want a pint?'

That was just his way. But my ma's father, Tom Kirwan, was on the run from the Free State Army and before that the British Army. In 2016 I was asked to do the Irish version of the TV show *Who Do You Think You Are?* It was a special episode for 1916, one hundred years of Irish Independence. They were looking at people in the public eye whose families were involved in the struggle.

They did all this digging and found everything they could about my grandfather. What they discovered was that he'd killed so many people it was probably best to leave our family out of the show. It was one of those things where it was better to pretend nothing had happened and move on.

He had a clatter of kids and I suppose it's much easier to go out and fight than it is to raise thirteen children, isn't it? When he was home, he'd always hide his gun in the pig shed because apparently a pig that has baby pigs is a lethal animal. It's like a miniature hippopotamus. And you don't mess with hippos – they look cute, but they'll eat you. Pigs have more or less the same reputation in Tipperary and the midlands. They were literally the Midland Piggy Militia, guarding guns for the IRA.

When I joined Sinn Féin, I did it because I think I was always looking for somewhere to belong. Once again, I was trying to find somewhere to fit in and something to do and something to be a part of, a recurring theme in my life. That nationalist way of thinking fills the gap in your life. It tells you, *No matter who you are, you're one of us.*

I got very involved in it very fast. It's my nature. There's only black and white, no grey area, with me. I'm either fully identifying with something and throwing myself into it, or I'm not getting involved with it at all. No half measures. I always need to have something to put my time into. And since I'd all the time in the world, that's how I ended up being full-time in Sinn Féin.

It started low-key enough, selling *An Phoblacht* and going to protests. And then before I knew it, I was wrapping a chain around myself outside the Department of Health because they weren't looking after drug addicts. Blocking up the Department of Justice, chaining the door shut to protest lack of rights for political prisoners. It all got a bit barmy really because I didn't have anything else going on.

This was '94 to '97, and at that time, being in Sinn Féin wasn't profitable or popular. Not like it is now. In fact, it was extremely unpopular. Everywhere you went the Garda special branch followed you. You got to know everyone in the special branch and they got to know you. Every time you left the building you were stopped and searched. When you went home you could see them outside your house. It was really intense. But it was easier than being at home.

It was great fun actually and I felt very at home in it. Before long I ended up working for Christy Burke, the first and only elected official of Sinn Féin at the time in Dublin City Council. He ran an advice centre but sometimes I'd be the only one there. People would come in saying they needed a house and I'd be like, 'Okay, okay. I'll write it down. I'll tell Christy.' I didn't have a clue but I did my best.

Then one day a woman came in and said she was being followed by the IRA and that they kept putting gas into her bedroom. She said she could prove it. So she opened a shoe-box she was holding and it contained a big shite.

She wanted me to take it away and get it sampled as proof the IRA were gassing her through her window. After that encounter, I didn't last in that office much longer but I still get on really well with Christy Burke. I love Christy Burke, he's a very good man.

One time we were outside Garda HQ on Harcourt Street, at the peak of the whole vigilante 'Get the drug pushers out of Dublin' movement. This was what I was really involved with, getting the drug pushers out, Concerned Parents Against Drugs and all that. Christy stood up and I think what he must have intended to say was, 'What we need is a huge electoral vote to push for change in the north inner city as we've been failed by everybody else.'

But what he actually said was, 'What we need is a huge electrical boat to fight for change in the north inner city as we've been failed by everyone else.' There was a sort of silence, and someone shouted, 'Go on, Christy.'

He never corrected it; he just left it at us needing a huge electrical boat – you can be guaranteed that at some point that evening someone was sitting somewhere wondering where we were going to get an electrical boat to sort out the heroin dealers.

At this point Sinn Féin is my full-time job, I'm there every day running Number 5 Blessington Street. It was the coldest building in the whole world. Then I moved over to do full-time work at the head office at 44 Parnell Square. At the time the big thing was protesting against the extradition of Tony Duncan back to the UK. He was an IRA guy from Finglas who was done for a series of attacks on the south coast of England where he attached small bombs to bicycles. Nobody was seriously injured.

Every couple of weeks we would go down to Green Street courts and protest and try to block the roads from the police vans, and one day I caused this full-on commotion. The following morning armed detectives came to the house and arrested me under Section 30, which is part of the Offences Against the State Act, and held me for suspected membership of an illegal organization. I spent one day in there getting questioned about everything.

Throughout that day in Raheny Garda station I worked out that this wasn't the life I wanted to have. Some people spend twelve years in custody and don't come to that realization, but it only took me twelve hours. Not long after, I took off for the States.

In Boston even more crazy stuff happened. We were all working illegally. The house we were staying in kept being broken into by a houseful of other Irish lads and they were wrecking it on us. One night they broke in and put hair remover on our eyebrows so none of us had any eyebrows for a few weeks. Another time they threw a pig's head into the front garden, copying something that had happened at a football match around the time. Terrible toxic masculinity it was.

There was a lot of drinking – a gang of twenty-something Irish lads let loose in Boston in the mid-90s, you can imagine. At one point we collected all the bottles in the house so we could get a bit of change from the bottle bank and buy something to eat. We spent it all on Oreos and more beer.

Close to when we were due to return to Ireland, we went on this big night out in Boston. We were in a taxi on the way back to the house when one of the lads decided to do a runner. We tried to talk him out of it until it dawned on us that none of us had any cash to pay the driver. We'd spent what we had in town and our latest pay cheques hadn't been cashed out yet. None of us had a penny.

We all legged it but one of the lads, Ger, fell asleep getting out of the taxi, conked out against the open door. So I had to go back and face the taxi man, who was going absolutely nuts looking for his money but I couldn't pay him, we only had our cheques. The solution I came up with was to break into the house where the other Irish lads lived, steal their television and give it to him as payment.

When I gave him the TV he kept roaring at me, saying, 'How do I know this thing even works, you cockavaroach! Fuck you, you cockavaroach Irish Paddy bastard!'

But then, suddenly, he just stopped roaring at me and drove off and that's when we realized he'd robbed Ger's passport out of his back pocket. What we didn't know then was that the police were on their way to the house to arrest us for wrecking it.

We went to a police station to file a missing report for the passport and somehow we managed to get the police report filed so we could get the passport back at some point, but we couldn't go back to the house – more police were there and they had Ger's name, because the taxi driver took his passport and gave it to them.

By this stage of the night one lot of coppers had been sent to arrest us for the state of the house and another lot were en route to the house with Ger's passport and a very angry Greek taxi driver in tow. Meanwhile, me and Ger had just filed a police report to try and get the passport back. It was a mad night and it got even madder.

Most importantly we had to get our cheques cashed; until we did that we'd no money. We went to a pub that used to cash them for us and take a 15 per cent tip but there was no one there. Ger found a fiver in his pocket, and we decided to buy two Starbucks Frappuccinos. The bill came to 5 dollars and 20 cents. We couldn't catch a break.

Eventually, through sheer shoe leather – walking all over the place to people's houses – we ended up getting enough money to ring a fella Ger knew in the GAA who said we could hide out in his house and he wouldn't say anything to the police about us being there. 'I won't say anything to the police and in the morning get lost.'

That was the deal. Grand. We got our cheques cashed, bought some frozen pizza and took it back to this man's house with a couple of beers. We stuck the pizza in the oven, opened the beers, but were so tired we fell asleep. When we woke up his oven was on fire. My first instinct was to try and stop the smoke alarms going off; I was more afraid of being in trouble than I was of burning the house down.

I'm wrapping wet towels around something that turned out to be the doorbell speaker and not the smoke alarm at all; he mustn't have had any smoke alarms because the oven was in flames and no bells went off. Ger managed somehow to put the fire out, and I don't know how he did it, but he did. We had to leave that house in the middle of the night because your man would've killed us, his whole kitchen was wrecked from the fire.

We split up then. I went to New York, got a job shovelling horse manure for a couple of weeks, then flew home.

When I got back Sinn Féin offered me a new role working with prisoners but I wasn't interested any more. That was it. It was all over.

It's a bit like that gag they have in *The Simpsons*: even if you can make a difference, you probably shouldn't. Best to mind your own business really, isn't it? Now, saying that, I've spent the last few years doing nothing but tell everyone my business and here I am sharing more of it. But there's a lot to be said for just getting on with your own life and staying out of everybody else's as much as you can.

15.

'Daddy.
Is. Dead.'

All his life we knew there was something very wrong with my da. He used to scream all night in his sleep at the top of his voice.

'*Fuck, fuck, fuck, fuck.*'

Every night. My ma couldn't share a bed with him because he'd fall asleep and thrash about screaming and kicking and punching. The nights we'd lie awake just listening to him screaming in his own bed.

We'd record him on tape recorders and play it back to him and he'd say, 'That's not me, that's the dog.' He really had no idea he was doing it even when we played it back to him. But why were we playing it back to him? We played it back to him to tell him to stop, but playing someone's terror back to them doesn't make them stop.

That was a brutal idea on our part, but we just wanted him to know it was real and we really desperately wanted it to end.

What was wrong? I would love to know. I'd still love to know that. No one had heard of PTSD but he had to have had it; it was like he was shell-shocked. Something horrific happened to him but I'll never know the answer to it. You don't get shell-shocked walking around Marino or Fairview.

The really good memories I have of me and my da are all pub-related. As a kid I'd often hear the lads talk about going to Howth with their families. They would go and walk the pier, or they'd walk the cliffs. The northside kids, that's where their parents would take them on the weekend: Howth, Portrane or Skerries.

Every so often, my old man would take me to Howth, but we'd just go to the pub, to the Cock Tavern. I have a strangely nice memory of being with him in the Cock Tavern on a very sunny day. He got me three sandwiches. Even back then I was thinking, 'This is ridiculous. I am a child.' He bought me a load of Cokes, and four of those war comics I was really into, so I must have been nine or ten.

It really was a beautiful sunny day. *So beautiful and sunny*, I thought to myself. *What a waste it would be to be outside walking in the sunshine. What a bleedin' waste.* Who needs fresh air and sunshine when you can sit in a pub with your da drinking Coke and eating sandwiches? It was just the two of us that day, no outside company. Usually when we'd go out to the pub some greasy old drunk would come over and I was left out. There was always someone who wanted to talk to him. But that day we sat there in the Cock Tavern, like two old men, reading our comics and newspapers. I was feeling slightly sick, overstuffed on cheese sandwiches. To this day I love that feeling. You know when people say, 'I stuffed my gob, I feel sick,' well, I don't know what they're complaining about, I still love that feeling.

That day with me da is one of my fondest memories, the only time I honestly didn't feel jealous of families walking around in the hills or going to football matches together. I was able to do all those things, but my old man never went with me. So this was a big day.

We didn't say anything to each other, not that I can recall. In fact, now that I think of it, it couldn't have been the Cock Tavern because the place had a video jukebox and Feargal Sharkey's 'A Good Heart' and Black's 'Wonderful Life' were playing on repeat. So it must have been 1985, when I was ten. Those songs played over and over and the two of us sat there eating our sandwiches and having the craic. Best day ever. Never had a day like that with him again until he was told he had cancer.

The first time my da collapsed in the house was around the time I was pulled in for questioning by the guards in Raheny, which is why I can pinpoint the time frame of it. I just thought the drink was finally getting to him. I didn't realize he had cancer, no one did.

After I got back from Boston and turned down the job with Sinn Féin, I had a series of terrible jobs. The worst job I ever did, in my life, was with an air-conditioning outfit down in Tipperary. I rang a friend, Fiona Browne, and said, 'Fiona, listen, I need to get out of this, I want to do something in performance, anything! Can you help?' I ran away from Tipperary in the middle of the night and Fiona helped me prepare to audition for the Gaiety School of Acting.

I started in the Gaiety in 1998. The year after, my da got sick. That was the first time I really got to know him, when he was in the hospital. It was also horrendous but, in a way – and I feel guilty about it even now, although I know I shouldn't – I remember that time fondly, my old man dying of cancer. That was when I got to know him, got to experience him not being pissed, got to have conversations with him. The hospital was a predictable environment; he wasn't one man at three o'clock and some other lunatic at four o'clock.

Addiction's a curse of a thing, though. When he was in hospital my da couldn't drink. When he was being discharged, he said to me, 'Oh, I have to go around and get something, this drink that I have to get, the hospital told me I have to get it.'

I was like, 'Go around where? What are you talking about?'

'Oh, just around here.'

He was hardly able to walk – he had to lean against the wall, he couldn't stay on his own feet because the tumours had gone into his brain and his balance was gone. We walked down the road and into this B&B. He looked kind of drunk though he wasn't; he was just messed up from cancer. He started winking and making faces at the man behind the desk saying, 'We need that drink,' as if your man was going to give him something. The guy just kicked us out and slammed the door in our face.

I don't know how I fell for it, why I believed him, I must have genuinely believed things had changed. Christ Almighty, the disappointment, standing there, so angry at him.

'Everything you're going through and everything you've been through and the first thing you want to do when you come out is have a fucking drink.'

In the end, my da died of a heart attack on top of cancer on top of really bad kidneys, on top of fucked-up lungs and a really bad flu. It was a brilliant multitasking death. He was fifty-eight years old.

At my da's funeral my ma insisted on talking, even though that was the priest's job – literally what he was there for.

Every so often during the service she'd stand up, wave wildly in the direction of the coffin, and put on her posh accent, the one she gets the minute a drop of wine has hit her lips, and at this point one or two drops had:

'Cancer came into our lives and stole Daddy. Daddy died. Poor Daddy. He was not feeling very well, and now he's dead. Daddy. Is. Dead.'

Father Maher was sitting beside me and kept whispering into my ear as she rambled on, 'She doesn't even have any notes!' This seemed to be what concerned him the most, that she'd no notes. Maybe she didn't have any notes but she had had three bottles of wine.

For the trip to the cemetery my ma wouldn't get into the family car to follow behind the hearse like a normal person. She insisted on sitting in the front seat of the hearse.

'I need to sit in the front with Daddy.'

All we had to do was drive half a kilometre to the cemetery, a kilometre at a push. But, no, it couldn't be that simple, she wanted to do a tour of Marino first.

'I want to see the church where I married Daddy.'

Then she wanted to see the old pub they used to run and then she had to see the first house we ever lived in. And behind us there's a massive line of cars and nobody knows where they're going. The poor undertaker, he's never, ever had a widow in the passenger seat giving him directions and asking him a million questions about who he is and where he comes from. Turns out he's a Protestant from Laois.

'A Protestant! A Protestant driving Daddy to his grave!'

Bikes have always been there for me, getting me out of the house and out of my head. After my da died I was very upset. Understandably, I suppose. Just very upset. Jason had just bought himself a new Vespa and he lived near me at the time. He told me to try out the Vespa, have a shot at it. It was the old type with the three gears on the handlebars.

I drove down Hollybrook Road on to the seafront and for the first time since my aul man died, I wasn't happy or sad, I was just in this really nice, non-feeling space, riding a bike in the sun. It was a huge relief. It was the first break from all the bullshit of cancer and the torture of watching someone you love just wither away. Seeing your father sober up and become a human being but a dying human being.

That day on Jason's Vespa was a huge moment, because that was the first time I recognized how much bikes had helped me over the years. In a weird way, the bikes I'd had had kind of been the reliable family I didn't have at home.

When my da died things got a lot better: no fighting any more, no one fuelling anyone else's drinking. To lose him was still very rough; I wasn't ready for it because you love your da and maybe he'd never talk to you or get engaged with you but the odd time, every so often, you'd just get an insight into the man and then that's when you'd know, *Oh yeah, there's a human banging around in there somewhere.*

And it's always small things that give you a glimpse of the human inside. I remember him telling me something that happened in school – he was looking into the sea and some lad pushed him over – and I had this feeling that I'd love to find that young lad and kick his head in. That's the thing, I suppose, I had feelings for the man.

And then there were other times. One night he was walking past my room and he came in and said, 'Fucking hard, isn't it?'

'What is?'

'Life, you know. Just fucking life.'

And I laughed!

Just laughed and he was like, 'Ahhhhh.' He closed the door and walked off.

I'll never forget it, just him expressing himself like that. It meant a lot to me that he would just come in and say that to me. Stand there and say, 'It's fucking hard, d'you know what I mean?'

When things were getting better for me, it was too late for him. What I'd always wanted the most, more than anything, was to be able to turn around to this big helpless child with a comb-over, who couldn't connect with anyone, and who screamed his way through his sleep every night, and let him know everything was going to be all right.

But it wasn't all right, and he died miserable. I wish I could have made him feel some sense of security before he died. Because that was something nobody in our house ever had.

My sister found security by building her family, but my way was to decide I'd never be part of a family ever again. I thought, *Okay, maybe there is a soulmate out there for everyone but, d'you know what, yours has four legs, wags its tail and shits outside. That's your soulmate.*

16.
Soulmates

For me a family was a house full of people you're desperate to get away from. When I was a kid I remember begging my parents to split up because of all the fighting and the drinking. They said, 'Oh no, we'll never do that, we're going to stay together because we love you so much.' I learnt to see love as a very dangerous trap.

Loving someone was something I was always very, very comfortable with, but as soon as they loved me back, I panicked, I couldn't take it, I was terrified they were going to tie me down. Terrified they would take something away from me, take whatever level of freedom I'd gained for myself, whatever sort of personal choice I had built up by having a job, by being independent.

I think that's why I've always been so attached to dogs, ever since I was a small boy putting straws on Tara's head. I trust them and they never take anything from me. All they want is their basic needs met, some grub, a walk and a cuddle. Growing up they were such an immense comfort to me, and they still are.

There's people who don't like dogs at all and I'll never understand it. And not only do they not like them, they spend their energy trying to keep them off beaches and out of parks. Like humans don't have enough room in the world, now we're trying to keep animals out of actual nature. Try and bring your dog on a holiday in this country or rent an apartment so you both have somewhere to live. You won't be able to do it.

It's always the same objection, isn't it? They're smelly. Everyone always says they're smelly. *You're smelly*. People are smelly. Look in your shower, look at all the crap you have to put on yourself to stop smelling like a turd.

If you went two to three months between grooms, I know nobody would even look at you. We are all hairless apes walking around, so get over yourself with your 'dogs are smelly' high and mighty attitude.

At least a dog has the decency to die when it's a teenager. You know what I mean? It won't turn around and start saying, 'I don't wanna be seen with you in public.' And before they hit puberty you can neuter your dog. You can cut their nads off and then say, there, that's that sorted.

Our last family dog was Saoirse. My sister and my ma drove up to Wicklow somewhere and bought Saoirse off a farmer. On the drive back he puked all over my sister in the car, so he got off to a great start. But Saoirse, he was the greatest animal. He was the most placid, lovely, friendly boy. He was another collie, like Skippy, they're great dogs. Saoirse was the dog that taught me dogs are absolutely 100 per cent better than human beings, no doubt about it. I was older than when I had Tara and I could really appreciate him.

He could do everything. I swear to God that dog could have done origami if you'd let him. He could play football; we'd play headers together down at the seafront and he never wanted or needed a lead. Completely reliable all the time and so restrained. Most dogs you say, 'D'you wanna go for a walk?' and they lose their minds. Saoirse would look at you as if to say, 'Sure, if it suits you.'

I used to run around St Anne's Park trying to get fit – I'm one of those people that has an on/off relationship with fitness – and this dog would have total patience with me, just do whatever I was doing, run, walk, run, walk. He lived to serve. All he wanted was to make people happy; he spent his whole day desperately trying to work out what would make me or anyone else happy.

He lived to a good age but his death was awful. I'll never forget the vet coming round and giving him the injection in our kitchen. It was the worst thing ever. I wasn't ready for that one. Everything about it was awful. Watching him not being able to walk any more. On his last day I remember sleeping on the kitchen floor with him – I wouldn't leave him on his last day. His nose was so grey and I could see how much he was trying to hang on. He was a silent battler, everything you want to be in your life, a stoic, silent servant of goodness. Then the vet put him in a plastic bag and threw the body in the boot. I'll never forget it.

I've two dogs now, Wendy and Stella, who I share with my ex-wife Elaine. Stella is a Staffordshire Terrier with an anxiety disorder and she's going bald. I've no idea why she's suffering from anxiety 'cause she's the most mollycoddled dog in the world.

At one point we tried her on a vegan diet, to see if her fur would grow back. People would be handing her treats and I'd have to say, 'Sorry, she's a vegan.' You'd want to see the faces looking back at me. 'She's a bleedin' wha'?'

Finally, I took her to this Polish lad who works specifically with bull breeds and he's brilliant but expensive. I've spent so much money on this dog, honest to God anyone else would have shot her by now but I love her, she breaks my heart. Oh, she breaks my heart. But she's really coming around, she's chasing squirrels with confidence now and getting playful again, the tail is up in the air and I'm so proud.

Dogs are there to remind us that the small stuff in our lives is the important stuff, they really are. You come home and they're like *Look what I did, look what I did, I did a shite, isn't it marvellous!*

And you think, *You know what, I love a shite too.* I love sitting on the loo for ages on my phone learning stuff while my legs go dead. You have to read on the jacks, don't you, or else your bum will know you're listening? My da used to head to the jacks with a newspaper and six or seven Benson & Hedges. It's the male yoga.

Dogs are great company. I could talk to Stella all day long. *So, what else did you do? You saw another dog? Well, that's only brilliant!*

And then you feed them the same food from the same bag every day and they can't believe what's happening. They think it's the best thing that's ever happened.

And they always know when you're in a bad way. Especially rescue dogs. I remember crying over a break-up once, my head in my hands. It didn't help that the break-up happened on Christmas Day. Each one of those things is awful enough on its own but combine them and you're into a full-scale meltdown. Lilo, my first ever rescue dog, came over and put her head in my lap. Somehow, they just know that you've saved them from death row, so they really look after your back.

*

Breaking up and getting back together and breaking up and getting back together, this same routine kept happening over and over again through my whole life.

It's a dysfunction, something broken in my head. That's what I've always thought.

Monogamy I have always tried at so hard and failed at so badly. I've never, ever been able to pull it off, even though I really was so in love with the people I was in relationships with. There was always something so good about the chase. Being in the chase I was happy. But once the relationship arrived or settled down, the panic started. Arriving into something always felt to me like I was back in the family dynamic I had always been trying so hard to escape. Somebody telling me they loved me always translated to me as 'I own you', and I didn't know how to shake that off, I couldn't reason myself out of it.

With girlfriends it was always that way. I'd be in these relationships where I loved someone, like desperately loved them and wanted to do really nice things with them and make them happy and all that stuff. Then, as soon as they said they loved me and were in it for me and only me I would freeze and think, that's not what I want.

The fact of the matter is I've blown up so many good relationships. I'm one of the luckiest people in the world in that every single person I've ever been with has been a really good person. Every woman I've been in a relationship with has always given me the 100 per cent I asked for and then couldn't understand why I couldn't give 100 per cent back. Could never understand why I was so flippant and easy about stuff.

Elaine is probably the single greatest person I've ever met. My relationship with her is the deepest friendship I've ever had and the best relationship I've ever had.

We have spent a huge chunk of our lives together and we got married. Fifteen years we were together overall, being so in love and great friends and fitting together so well. Still, even with Elaine, I couldn't grasp the simplest concept of someone being in it just for me and me giving her back the 100 per cent she was giving me. Such a simple thing, such a reasonable request, just asking for what everybody else has.

I could never understand why that kept happening; all I had was my own pop psychology, my head telling me it was because of my parents. That was all I had to go on: *Nothing works out because of my background.* And, of course, there's a model we inherit of how romantic relationships are supposed to work, that model only has two people in it and I never really questioned it.

Sometimes in relationships someone would say to me, 'How would you like it if I was with someone else?' and there was always a voice in the back of my head that was curious, wondering, 'Oh, yeah, who's that then, this person that you like? Are you into them? Do you have a closeness with someone, an affection for someone? Are you hanging out with someone who's not just a friend, but it's not a relationship either?'

Of course, that wasn't the response they were looking for and I didn't fully understand my reaction myself; it always confused me, that lack of jealousy.

Two years ago I started talking to a girl called Danielle that I met through the tattoo scene. She's from Canada and such an unusual alternative character, she seems like an alien from another planet to most people. She won't mind me saying that; she's proud of it. Danielle is into so many things: kinks and whips and chains and rubber knickers and plastic socks, glass dildos, inflatable donkey dicks hanging off the roof, the lot.

She's also polyamorous. Now, until that moment I had never heard that word, or if I had it hadn't registered with me. I'd heard of swingers, which is all about sex. And I'd heard of polygamists, which is some dude with loads of wives who aren't allowed to do very much except have children. It was always tied to some odd religious stuff in Utah and very male-focused, like most religious stuff.

When Danielle told me she was polyamorous I thought she meant a casual sex thing, and although I've done them, one-night stands aren't really my scene, I've never really had the head for them. But Danielle explained that polyamory means that you can be with someone, love someone and share your life with someone and not get involved in the escalator of relationships. She explained that most regular relationships are polyamorous, that it's only the romantic relationship we confine to two people.

For instance, if you have a kid, you love that kid with all your heart. And then if you have another kid, you don't have to take love off the first kid, to give it to the second kid. You just love both your kids. Same with your friends. You love all your friends. You love all your pets. So why can't you love all your partners?

As long as people are honest with each other it can work, because it's always the dishonesty that destroys relationships. I've cheated on people instead of being honest with them. I hate the fact that I did it, but I did. Not sure there's that many people who can say they haven't.

People think it's all about sex but they're confusing it with open relationships. Polyamory is primarily about intimacy. A lot of polyamorous people are completely asexual, they don't like having sex at all. They just want intimate partners they can share time with that they don't share with anybody else.

Some polyamorous people are demisexual, which means emotional attachment is more important to them than sexual attraction. And some people are polysaturated, which means they have enough partners and don't have the time for any more. (I can't even believe I'm throwing around these terms. These are words that two years ago I would've said, 'Oh, would you get over yourself, you!')

Look at how many divorced people are raising kids and hate each other. These are people who got on to the relationship escalator, moved in together, got a house together, realized they hated living together and instead of just changing their relationship they broke the whole relationship down. *We have to split up now. We have to sell the house, sell the car, fight over who gets to talk to the kids.*

Wait, why can't you just still be in a relationship together and raise the kids and it be okay? The whole living together thing didn't really work, but everything else is all right.

You know, it doesn't have to go one way. It can go any direction, at least I think it can. I feel it can, and it works for me. I mean, I'm reasonably new to what is, I suppose, for want of a better word – and I cringe even saying this – the 'lifestyle'.

Lifestyle isn't the right word, and I don't feel like I'm part of a community either. What I am is someone who is able to be completely in love with different people at the same time and is able to cope with the idea of someone saying, 'I love you' and 'I also love this other person.' That feels so much more at home in my heart, it doesn't make me panic. It doesn't feel like ownership any more because it's not all on me. I'm not all they need, and I don't have to try and fulfil every need they have.

Nobody can be everything you're looking for in a

relationship. That's a lot of pressure. People expect to find someone who looks a certain way, is funny and compassionate, spontaneous, and good with finances, responsible and carefree. Nobody is all these things, so get three or four people! Love them all! Love the shit out of them! Love them till your ass falls off!

Before, I always felt like such a huge disappointment to people because it didn't worry me if they wanted to connect with someone else, hang out with other people. The thing was, I wanted to hang out and connect with other people, that was important to me. I grew up in a house where no one was connected to anyone at all; I wasn't connected to my ma, I wasn't connected to my da, I didn't know my sister, there were six strangers in the house. The booze was first, the patients were second and the dog was third. In that house I was just completely loose and disconnected.

Now I can go and make connections with people and sometimes that connection is a nice chat and a cup of coffee and sometimes that connection is physical. Maybe that connection will go on to become a relationship; being polyamorous does not exclude connecting with a constant partner and having a family like Kelly and I are doing. And out of respect for Kelly's privacy, I'm going to leave it at that.

There's no rules other than respect in polyamory, so for the first time in my life everything feels so accessible, I've found a place that I can flourish in. Love always felt like such a sacrifice before, even though I had such fantastic women in my life, most of whom I'm still good friends with.

Which reminds me . . . in conversations with the teenagers and young people on the set of *The Young Offenders* sometimes they'll ask if I've any advice on lads. The one thing I always say is: *Never, ever, go out with a lad who says his ex is crazy.* Especially don't go near him if he says all his exes are crazy because the only thing they have in common is him. Lads who like their exes are a safer bet, even though people think it's the other way around.

'He still talks to his ex? Well, I'm not having that.'

It's the other way around. If he still respects and likes his exes that's a good thing. If he's saying all his exes are crazy whackjobs that's a big red flag, that's what you need to look out for.

To some extent you do have to come out as polyamorous, especially to yourself, but it's never going to be the same as being a gay person; you don't get vilified or bullied by society, nobody is going around saying, 'Jaysus. Imagine if you were someone who fancied FOUR people.' It's not the same, no matter what anyone says, there's no one out there battering polys for being poly, especially not on the North Strand where I am now.

It's not the same, but there is a coming-out process to it, an acceptance process from yourself to yourself, and I'll be eternally grateful to Danielle for helping me. (And I'd like to thank her for getting me into all of this. It's just amazing that one person could show me the road that's helped me find so much out about myself.)

If you take anything from this, the one thing I'd say is the main point of polyamory isn't sex. The main attraction of it for me is that it's allowed me to find my way to a place where I can love and be loved and not be in a panic about it, not be worried that I'm going to let people down, because I've screwed up a lot of relationships in the past.

I might screw up another one but I don't think I will.

I wish I'd discovered it earlier, but you can't do 'what ifs' when you're forty-eight years old. You'd only spend the second half of your life thinking about how you screwed the first half up and I'm more than halfway done, best case scenario.

17.
Stand-up

John Lynn used to have a great joke about life in stand-up along the lines of, 'Well, comedy, it's tough, it's hard to make a name for yourself and start filling rooms. Sometimes the money isn't great, but like, the hours, you just can't beat the hours.' And that's true. You're working real hard for one hour a day and the rest of the time you're driving.

We never see ourselves as drivers, but that's what we are. You get into your car, you drive three to four hours, you deliver jokes instead of a parcel and then you drive home. That's what you do – you deliver jokes.

I started doing stand-up because Jason kept telling me I should do it and because I felt like I could do it, not 'cause I wanted to do it. There were clubs, there were opportunities, and you always made a couple of quid. At the same time I was doing the clubs I was a motorbike courier, which was the perfect job to go with it. Everyone needed a guy on a bike back then, people couldn't just email everything to each other.

This was before the internet, so to let people know about

my gigs as I was motoring around I'd bring my posters and put them up all over the lampposts, over the big gig posters and the 'Post No Bills' signs. They were such complementary jobs: do a gig, get a courier job, stick up some posters, do another gig, get another courier job.

Stand-up was easier when I started. Now a lot of the stand-ups from back in the day, if they're reading this they will say, 'What do you mean it was easier? There was no scene, there was no comedy scene.' I know. That's why it was easier. I could literally go into a gig, into a venue, get up on the stage – or even just stand up at the top of the room in a pub – and start telling jokes. I didn't have to audition or learn lines. I just had to talk for ten or twenty minutes. They'd pay us thirty quid for that. Even if it was just to make us stop, we got something for it.

There used to be about twelve working stand-ups in the country and now there's 12,006. It was a harder time to find places to gig, there were fewer clubs, but if you found a place to gig and you went down well you could gig there all the time.

Now everywhere is full up because there's so many stand-ups. You walk into a place, and you say you want to practise your material and build up your ten or twenty minutes and they say, 'Sure, no problem, come back in seven or eight months.' Seven or eight months later you get a five-minute slot, and you have to wait another five months to do it again.

So, you're not getting stage time, you're not getting an opportunity to get better and be good. What happens then is cliques form and people who can't get gigs set up their own nights and give all their friends gigs and so you've got entire comedy clubs populated by bog standard material. We were lucky we never had any of that.

Nobody gets paid for anything now. And you have to market yourself online. If I'd had to do all that online work when I started, nothing would have happened for me. I didn't get into 'the arts' because I wanted a job where I had to work hard; the appeal for me was that it looked like a very handy number. There's not exactly a huge artistic integrity to that but that's the way it was.

I'm terrified of work. I hate lifting an arse or an elbow. Always have, still do. I am literally that person who if I had to walk to the bed, I'd lie on the floor. So the idea that you could walk into town in the early noughties, get on stage having not even known you were going to do a gig when you left your gaff, and get thirty pounds to drink for the night was just amazing. A very liberating feeling.

One thing the internet has absolutely ruined is how much obnoxious money you used to get paid for doing ads. After the Gaiety I signed with the agent Fiona Byrne. She called her agency 'Tongue Tied', because both me and this fella called Ruben that she represented had tied tongues. She got me into an audition for a Guinness ad, and much like the Channel Four show I'd do many years later, it's one of the only Guinness ads nobody remembers.

Everybody remembers the great Guinness ads – the Dancing Man and the settling pints, the lad on the surfboard, the white horses coming through the sea. But the fella running into a pub full of people cheering, no one remembers that one. That was me! The set-up was that I was wearing all blue and listening to a match on a small transistor radio held to my ear, heading towards the Windjammer pub on Townsend Street. I run into the pub, kick the door open just as the transistor radio is telling me my team has scored a goal.

Jumping round like crazy I suddenly stop because I've noticed that everyone in the pub is wearing red. It's obvious I've walked into a rival bar, and I back out all paranoid and sketchy. That was the ad, and I was paid 4,000 pounds which was sensational, outrageous money at the time.

By some weird twist of fate (or accounting error), the film company paid me four grand and so did the ad agency. I'd been paid 8,000 pounds for a day's work – I couldn't believe it! Fiona rang one of them up and said, 'PJ has been paid twice.' One of them sent me an email saying, 'Please put the money back in the account.' I went straight out and bought a motorbike instead.

I was doing a bit of stand-up then in the clubs and won the Jammy Bastard Award that year and got a big pot of jam for being such a jammy bastard and getting paid twice.

I wasn't making a living from stand-up yet. At this stage, in my early twenties, it was more like a cash subsidy. Full-length shows weren't something I even thought about, it didn't seem remotely likely that anyone was ever going to pay me to do an hour-long set.

As with the acting, there was all this pressure for Irish stand-ups to go abroad. 'Oh, you should go to Manchester or Edinburgh every year. You should conquer New York.' My attitude has always been, 'Conquer Leinster before New York.' At least bank some level of national success before packing your bags and heading off into the big bad world.

I looked to my idols, Pat Shortt and Tommy Tiernan, these big names with big careers in Ireland who didn't go anywhere else. Tommy's changed that now, but back then, that's how I saw him. And that's what I wanted. I don't even like holidays very much. When I started to tour around the country I went home to Dublin every single night.

I'm a very competitive person. If I was ever on a bill with anybody else, if I was ever on a line-up with anybody else, if I was doing festival shows where you get four or five people and you all have to do your best twenty minutes or your best twenty-five minutes, if I wasn't hands-down, absolutely the greatest person on that night, I would be raging with myself.

I didn't think, *D'you know what, I had a good gig but that person was better.* No. The way I saw it was that everyone was shit at this stupid thing. So if someone was better than me it meant I was shittier than shit.

So, at the end of every single gig, I would have to get the biggest cheer or the biggest round of applause. I had to, I needed that. Walking off stage I needed to have a genuine feeling that the people that night thought it was the funniest show they had ever, ever, ever seen.

Otherwise, it would all feel like a total and utter disappointment. I've never been a great joke writer, but I know I can tell a story and nobody works harder on the stage than I do. A lot of comedians have to work a lot harder to be able to tell a story as well as I can.

Take Neil Delamere, for example. Neil is a brilliant joke writer, he's a joke machine. And his ambition – you can actually hear his ambition. He has put in the work. He has the jokes, he's prepared. That's the bit I'm not so good at.

But when I get on stage, I know I'm as good as anyone. This sounds quite egotistical, but whether it's Chris Rock or Jerry Seinfeld or some experimental Edinburgh wanker, I'm going to blow them off the stage. That's something I worked out pretty quickly and I'd always look at other comedians when they were getting on stage and think to myself, *What are you even doing here?* So, yeah, I've a competitive edge.

And that's what I enjoyed about stand-up and got out of it, that feeling of, *At least, I'm really good at this.* Being good at something and getting paid for it felt great. But I was never actually into comedy. That's the whole point. Still to this day, people say something like, *Have you seen the new* – I don't know – *Knicker McDickers Netflix special?* No, I haven't. I don't have a clue who these people are, and I wouldn't go to a stand-up gig, not even if you threatened to shoot me in the bollox.

18.
Stand down

The years started to tick by, and what was once exciting but never fun was getting a bit depressing because I wasn't making a living from it. I was only just really scraping by, and you can only tell yourself being good at something is enough for so long. It's not enough.

The gigs were going well but I was getting frustrated. I was never afraid to experiment, but in a lot of venues the stand-ups would want a microphone and they'd stand at the corner of the bar on a crate, and I didn't like it, it was too confining. Anyway, I didn't need the microphone, I'm naturally a loud person, so I'm able to talk really loud and project myself. Bit of a noisy pig really.

I always wanted to make things natural. I didn't want to stand there with a mic; the gigs needed to feel like you were listening to your friend telling you his latest crazy escapade. And I had to be the punchline of all my jokes. That was important for me because I think that's Irish humour.

Now, I'm in danger of losing half the crowd here when I talk about the risks of being cancelled. I'm not saying, 'You can't say anything now,' so bear with me. When it comes to stand-up, you used to be able to get on stage, say something that was risky and if the audience didn't like it, you would be rewarded with silence. It wasn't, 'I'm gonna make sure you never work again.' You would get silence and then you realized, 'Oh, that was a bit insensitive. I'm not gonna do that again.' There was more room to make mistakes, to fail. Times have changed. Some of the stuff I was doing back then I'd never do now. As you get older what you find funny changes. What your audience finds funny changes. The more you learn along the way the more you evolve. Suffice it to say my last show was called 'Dickhead'.

Without on-the-job training it's a lot harder now for a stand-up to blow the roof off the place. As I mentioned already, there's the scarcity of spots to trial material, and as well as that, there's less focus on being funny for the sake of being funny. People blowing the roof off is much rarer now than it used to be. Joe Rooney told me once, 'If you can't be funny, be interesting.' And it's like since the day he told me that everybody has decided to be interesting.

Joe Rooney is a very funny comedian, so he never had to take the interesting route – he's a brilliant stand-up – but he was obviously observing the scene, because as soon as he said it I noticed there were a lot of interesting comedians around but nobody who'd make you wet yourself laughing. Now everybody seems to have a message of some sort.

At this point I was gigging for nearly ten years. Started doing the sketch shows with Jason, went to the Gaiety, graduated and gave up acting immediately. Then I hit the comedy circuit doing the clubs, comedian-for-hire slots at events, a tour sponsored by Carrolls cigarettes and bits at the

Kilkenny Cat Laughs Comedy Festival, but never getting main slots. It was getting very, very frustrating.

Everybody cared more about the international acts, which I've never understood because Irish people love Irish acts. You bring international acts to Irish festivals and some of these stand-ups, they have great reputations among international festivals – 'You have to see this comedian, they're incredible, their take on socialism in the twenty-first century is just sooooo spot on.' Deco and Dave and Debbie down at the comedy festival in the Iveagh Gardens, they don't give a shit. They want to have a laugh. They see right through you, you pretentious knob, and they know you're not being funny.

The reality was I was still supplementing this 'career' with other jobs and had been for a bit too long at this stage. Looking to the future, did I really want to be hauling my arse around the place at fifty or sixty, doing open spots?

Naturally, you start thinking, *What am I doing with my life?* One of my cousins was very successful and my ma made some comment about how well he was doing, about how much better he was doing than I was. It wasn't nice to hear and I was a bit taken aback but I couldn't say she was wrong.

The *Herald* used to have all these jobs on the back page, and I'm looking at them thinking, 'I'm not qualified for anything. I've no trade. I've supplemented my stand-up income for years working in chemical plants, working in air-conditioning, being a courier, working on building sites, but I've no trade. On a building site I've absolutely no skills. I'm just the guy everyone shouts at to pick things up and put things down.'

I remember thinking, *I gotta get outta here, I have to clear my head. Whatever money I have, I'm just gonna take it, get on a bike and go missing.* This was 2004. I decided I'd get on my bike and travel all around Europe. The plan was to ride the bike until

I ran out of money. The hope was that by the time I came home I'd have made some decisions about how to manage my life. Ridiculous. Running away from my problems.

As I was getting ready to leave, I got a phone call from a guy called Liam McGrath.

'Listen, we're making this hidden camera show for RTÉ, would you be interested?'

'No, I wouldn't. I'm going away on my bike. I've been doing this stand-up lark for ten years now and I haven't gotten anywhere.'

'Oh, okay, well, look, we're doing it anyway. Thanks for taking the call.'

So I got on the bike and drove around. I went down to Cherbourg and through Brussels, Amsterdam, out around Germany through Hamelin, the Pied Piper town (based on a true story by the way; the kids didn't go off dancing, but they did disappear). Right down through Dresden and all through Eastern Europe, down through Kosovo and Bosnia as far as the Albanian border. The Albanian guard looked at my bike and said to me, 'If you go in there, they're gonna take it off of you.' Albania had just undergone a period of anarchy a few years beforehand, so it was really unsettled at the time. From Montenegro I got a ferry to Italy and at this stage I was running out of money and had to make my way home.

I drove through Italy, France, all around the coast, went to the Basque Country in Spain, and eventually I came home seven weeks after the day I left and without a pot to piss in. All I had was my bike and my jacket, nothing else. So I rang Liam McGrath on the off-chance and said, 'You're not still looking for someone for this hidden camera show, are you?'

'Actually, we are. One of the cast just left in a rage.'

Brilliant.

19.
Naked Camera

I didn't think *Naked Camera* was going to be any good. It's RTÉ and it's comedy so, very likely, it won't be any good, but my philosophy in comedy is, if we can just make something that's not total and utter shite it'll be worthwhile doing it. And I had to do something, I was at a serious loose end.

First, I had to audition. How do you audition for a hidden camera show? It's not like I could go into a room full of directors and read a few lines, you know?

They asked me to meet them in the car park of Phibsboro Shopping Centre. The day before they asked me what I wanted to do and I was like, 'Oh my God, I don't know.' I couldn't think of anything, not one single thing. The only thing that came to mind was to print up some fake cash and I'd try to buy things with it.

So they printed up some cash and handed me a bag with a hidden camera in it in the shopping centre car park. They gave me a jumper to put on and I walked into Lappin Real Estate Agents and tried to buy a house with a bag of counterfeit cash. That was my audition and it ended up being the very first sketch, 'Jumperman', broadcast on *Naked Camera*.

When we did the reveal, your man in the real estate agency said to me, 'You're such a good actor. My God.' He was totally bought in. 'You had the shaky hands and all going on, you know, like a proper drug addict.'

That wasn't good acting, I was just really nervous, but it went well and I had a feeling straight away that there was something in it. I watched the teaser trailer that the other lads had done, and I remember thinking, much as I did with *Young Offenders* years later, 'There might be something in this, this could have some kind of impact.'

Naked Camera only happened because of a Dublin gangster. Liam was making documentaries for Prime Time, and he'd hired all this hidden camera equipment to film some gangster out in Clondalkin. But when he was sitting there filming didn't your man spot the camera, pull out a gun and threaten to shoot him?

Liam got out of the situation, but he was left with all this gear he'd spent a load of money on. He wanted to do something with it, but he didn't want to get killed, he'd just had a kid. So he thought, 'Well, if I can't film criminals, maybe I'll make a comedy show instead, at least with comedy nobody tries to murder you.'

That's literally how it happened. So, if a gangster didn't nearly kill a man there wouldn't have been a Jake Stevens, there wouldn't have been a Dirty Aul Wan or a Jumperman, which is bizarre when I think about it.

The other thing about *Naked Camera* is timing, the early to mid-noughties was the only time we could have made that show. People still had a lot of memories and affection for *The Live Mike*, the first hidden camera show that was made in

Ireland. We even had some of the same crew that worked on that show, like the sound man, Joe Dolan. And people weren't yet walking around with cameras on their phones.

People often say to me, 'Would you not bring back the Dirty Aul Wan? Would you not bring back Jake Stevens?' I can't! It wouldn't work. It just wouldn't work now. TikTokers, YouTubers, Instagram influencers, they're all out there doing sketches. Everybody's got a camera on their phone.

As soon as something weird happens in the world now, people automatically think, 'Who's looking at me? Who's filming me?' In 2004, 2005 and 2006 people didn't think like that, they just thought, 'Here's a halfwit that needs a bit of attention.'

What I always say about doing *Naked Camera* is that it renewed your faith in people. No matter what the problem, people would always try and help you. They'd be very annoyed about it but they would try and help you. So you'd go over to some guy and go, 'I'm after losing my monkey.'

'What the hell are you doing in town with a monkey for Jesus' sake! I've got somewhere to be! Where did you last see it?'

Now he's looking for the monkey with you though he's really annoyed with you because he didn't want to look for a monkey; he wanted to go and get a chicken roll. Amazing. That was my favourite thing about it.

Looking back, obviously there was a fair amount of mad stuff going on when I was a kid and a lot of big characters around. The weird thing is that they're not actually the people I based my *Naked Camera* characters on. Well, none of the ones named in this book inspired the characters, and none of the men who lived in our house did either.

If I'm to analyse why that is I'd say it's probably because none of them were obnoxious or cruel on purpose; they were just eccentric, addicted or screwed up. For all their faults, they were never boring. Whereas each *Naked Camera* character is either a horrible person or an eejit. There were no good guys, and I suppose doing them was a bit of a purge for me. They were a culmination of lots of different people I'd met along the way.

Jake, for instance, is an egomaniac. Jake can do no wrong.

'Hamlet once wrote a sonnet –' he might say.

'No, Jake,' you might cut in, 'it was Shakespeare who wrote the sonnets.'

'Well, now, we're going to have to agree to disagree on that one.'

Jake will always think you're the idiot, but he won't push it, you're not worth his time.

The Dirty Aul Wan is essentially a pervert, a sexual predator of sorts. And then there's like the Jumperman who's quite obviously a thief and a moron and doesn't want to do anything by the law. The only one that's any way decent is the Taxi Man, who's kind of an alien really. But even he is really self-centred. No matter what you say when you get into his taxi, he's taking you where he wants you to go and you're essentially at his mercy.

'No, we're not going there, I'll take you where I want you to go.'

By getting to parody them I was getting my own back on the sorts of people who had tortured me over the years. Self-important bores – you know them well, we've all met them. It's like a gas is seeping out through their nipples and it tortures you. Puts you to sleep while at the same time has you wracked by physical pain. And all they're doing is talking: *'Wah wah wah wah wah wah wah wah wah.'*

It didn't take me long to realize that when you tell people about a prize arsehole their ears prick up. People get really into it because everyone's been the victim of an arsehole. Everyone's listened to some egomaniac bragging about how amazing he is. Or met some gobshite who wants to talk about his sexual conquests. Or had some delusional halfwit bang on about himself in a self-congratulatory way.

All male examples because I think it's generally blokes who go on about how great they are. Women can be annoying too, of course. But the women I've met who are annoying are annoying in a different way. They're less likely to be singing their own praises from the rooftops – that's definitely more of a male thing.

We worked out that we did, in total, something like 760 sketches over three series. Only a tiny proportion of them made it into the show. Some of the best ones never made it in because people in Ireland are never where they're supposed to be. So, many people were like, 'I can't sign the release form, I'm on the dole, I'm not supposed to be working.' Or 'I can't sign the release form, I'm not supposed to be in the bookies, I told the missus I was down the supermarket.' But it added to the fun and flavour of the gig. It was great craic making that show.

For the three years I did *Naked Camera* it kind of took over my entire life. We did the *Naked Camera Live* tour: me, Maeve Higgins and Patrick McDonnell. Except it wasn't *Naked Camera Live*, it was just the three of us doing individual standup, so after that I decided to do my own gigs because I realized I could sell them out on my own. I didn't know how long all this would last, so I wanted to make a career for myself out of it and I wanted to make money.

Before *Naked Camera* I was a fella who did a bit of stand-up and had a decent reputation in the clubs. There were conversations with TV companies the odd time, with very little ever coming out of it. You'd do bits here and there, but nobody knew your name and you never made any money. So, to go from that to being asked to do every single thing, it was such a turnaround.

RTÉ, in their wisdom, were asking me for new show ideas all the time, and every year I'd write down some new ideas and every year they'd come back and say, 'Can we do *Naked Camera* again?'

There was a great sketch going around at the time taking the piss out of us all – me, Neil Delamere, Jason Byrne and Des Bishop. In the sketch we're all in RTÉ pitching our new ideas and they knock them all down and say, 'What about *Naked Camera Four*?' APPROVED. 'What about *The Panel* again?' APPROVED. 'What about *Anonymous* again?' APPROVED.

In fairness, at that time, Monday night comedy on RTÉ Two was really working. It was a big night. It was kind of the last of those nights when people would sit in and watch terrestrial TV on purpose. There was *The Panel*, *Podge and Rodge* and whatever Des Bishop was up to.

Everyone loves to say RTÉ wouldn't give anyone a chance, but at that time RTÉ were giving people chances left, right and centre. The TV people were going to the clubs, giving everyone shots. It's hard, though, to come up with good concepts for comedy shows; a lot of it is luck. RTÉ got stuck flogging to death anything that worked.

We went out and tried to do a *Naked Camera Four* because they kept asking us to. We got caught every single time. We tried one sketch where we were told, 'Don't worry, he'll never know, he's been living in Australia for the last four years and he's only after getting back last week and your show hasn't been on for six months and he won't have a clue who you are.'

He opened the door and he goes, 'Hey, PJ, what's the craic?' Someone had sent him a DVD for Christmas. So it was just ridiculous. We couldn't get away with anything.

When *Naked Camera* came out that first year it was a weird experience. The first series aired and for the first time ever, I started getting recognized on the street. Even though I'd been doing stand-up for ten years the perception was, 'Jesus, he came out of nowhere.'

The first year when people recognized me it was, 'There's that fella off the TV.' The second year it was, 'There's Jake Stevens,' and the third year, 'There's PJ Gallagher.' So it took the three series for people to work out who I was and that just led to a whole new world. It was just bananas. This mad trip had begun.

Suddenly, every venue I wanted to play would have me and everywhere I played was full. People were actually listening to my set because they'd come to see me and wanted to listen to my set. I started getting offered Vicar Street gigs on my own, being asked to headline festivals, touring to big venues like the Cork Opera House and earning decent money doing it. I'll never forget walking down Thomas Street to go to my own gig at Vicar Street and seeing a fellow outside going, 'Anyone buying or selling the tickets to PJ Gallagher. Anyone buying or selling tickets?'

DVDs were huge business then and I was one of the first Irish comedians to sign to Universal, if not the first. If you're of a certain vintage you'll remember HMV on Grafton Street, with the famous sign of the dog with the gramophone;

it was the main place for CDs and DVDs and it was where all the big stuff happened, all the album signings, everything. When my first DVD came out at Christmas 2007 I went in to have a look. I just wanted to see it on the shelf in this iconic place in Dublin. Having a DVD on that shelf, alongside all those other comedians, just being in the mix, you kind of felt like you'd made it.

Still, I couldn't get too cocky. One day I was standing in the queue to pay for something and there was a woman in front of me with Des Bishop's, Tommy Tiernan's and my DVD in her hand. Kind of cool, I was chuffed. Then one of the sales assistants came up to her with Neil Delamere's DVD and said, 'I found the one you were looking for.' The woman goes, 'Oh brilliant,' takes it off her, hands her my DVD and says, 'You can put that one back.'

That DVD made me so much money – even by today's standards it would be considered a lot – but nobody buys DVDs any more. Another way for stand-ups to make money that's been wiped out. Netflix special? Not a chance you'd see anything like the kind of money we were making then.

I'd only ever wanted to be good at something. I never expected to be very successful at stand-up, so that was a big surprise and there was plenty to keep me busy. I also started doing a lot of corporate gigs for big companies like Bank of America, standing up and chatting to a load of suits for twenty minutes while they eat their turkey and ham dinner. Corporates are so well paid but, by Jesus, they're so hard. It's all you can do to stop yourself saying, 'Think of the money' into the microphone. They are joyless, soulless, awful experiences. But you do them.

It was a period where I was making so much money, I didn't know what the money was for. These remittance slips would arrive, and I wouldn't know what gig it was I'd been paid for. Amazingly, it's all gone now.

The thing is, after riding the wave of a big success like *Naked Camera*, you get what you want but you still have to live the rest of your life. It's like, right, I've ticked that box, now what am I going to do? Where do I go from here?

20.
The Young Offenders

After the Gaiety I didn't really pursue acting work because auditions were a nightmare. I didn't mind doing the audition itself, it was the fact that you had to go and beg people to give you work, beg people to give you a job that could last for a day or six weeks max and then you mightn't get another one ever again. Spending the rest of your life auditioning for all these parts with the odds majorly stacked against you. Pretty much straight away I'm thinking acting is a terrible way to make a living.

Also, everybody was always telling you, 'Oh, if you wanna make a living as an actor, you have to go to England.' Really? Oh well. I'd rather iron my own tits than go to England. I would never do it. Or go to America. *America? Are you mad? People can't even understand what I'm saying in Kerry.*

I knew I was never going to be the romantic lead in any of these things. I'm more likely to get the part of a drug dealer or a criminal or a potato-headed monster than I am the heroic lead in a Hollywood movie. It's not going to happen. You have to become sort of realistic about your abilities and handicaps.

How you look, or how you're perceived to look, is so important and it almost doesn't matter what your ability is; you have to be what they're looking for before you even walk into the room. They have an image in their head. You can do the best audition in the world, you can blow the room apart, you can have them laughing or crying or feeling deeply about something, but if you're not what they're looking for, that's it. If the director or casting director is looking for a six-foot good-looking dude with blond hair and a nose ring and a mickey that goes down to his knee, the guy who fits the bill is getting the part.

That's what's so frustrating about acting and there's only so much 'Ah well, at least I know I did a good job' to get you through all the frustration. If you're a full-time actor, you still have to pay your bills and it's almost impossible. The number of roles I can do are so limited. This head is Fairview Park, not Notting Hill. No one is looking at this potato-head and saying, 'Let's cast him alongside Julia Roberts in a middle-aged comedy tragedy where he dies and she's heartbroken.' Julia Roberts is never going to be heartbroken over a head like mine, it's not a plausible scenario for a movie.

Still, I've always liked acting and it's something I've always wanted to do. I've just never exactly had the mental toughness, the resilience to keep getting turned down at auditions. (These days you don't even go to auditions. You just record yourself in your own kitchen against a white wall and send it in. So you get to fail miserably into your iPhone.) Trying to make a living from acting is just too much rejection to bear and I don't need to welcome that much rejection into my life, especially when I have the option to go on the radio every day or make up a few jokes.

The Young Offenders came along by pure chance because no

matter how many times I'd tell people I was interested in acting they'd look at me, baffled, as if I was in a carpenter's workshop asking for a roast chicken. They'd go, 'Oh, good for you,' and then make faces at each other. The minute I'd leave I guessed they'd be shaking their heads and saying to each other, 'Is he still going on about the acting? After all these years?'

Even if that's not true, that's exactly how it's always felt because I never get considered for acting roles. A few times I was offered roles without an audition. One was for a character called Fat Barry, a mentally challenged lad who spent his time outside off-licences buying drink for underage kids and got accused of a crime he didn't commit. When they rang me about it, they said, 'We think we have something that's perfect for you.' Right. Thanks a lot. Needless to say, I passed that one up.

So I never expected to land a role in *The Young Offenders*. I just got a call one day from the director, Peter Foott, who wanted me to play a drug dealer, which of course is the exact right fit. When I turned up to the audition, he showed me the trailer. The whole thing was practically finished, except for the bad guy because they hadn't been able to cast him. Watching the trailer, I knew straight away this was going to do something, that it was brilliant. It was just such a good feeling, and I threw myself into the audition – knowing that I could be a part of it was genuinely exciting. Whatever Peter said, I tried to make it bigger and better. For the first time in any audition I've ever done, before I left the room I knew I had the part.

It really was the *Thomas the Tank Engine* of comedy movies, the little movie that could. It was such a small production, the same woman doing my hair was catering the lunches, that'll tell you the size of the production.

For the film I had to get my head shaved down the middle and walk around Cork like that for a week; it was the strangest look ever. One night I was talking to a fella in a chipper and I took my hat off – you just forget, you've got this ridiculous haircut.

'How are you getting on these days? You're not doing much of the touring. It must be tough enough in the comedy business, is it?'

Clearly, this fella thought the stress of working in comedy had made me bald.

When the film wrapped there were so many premieres, which I did not know anything about. I'd always thought a premiere happened once, it was a first-night-ever thing. I didn't realize movies travelled the world doing a lot of first-time-evers. We had one in Cork and two in Dublin and then the Galway Film Fleadh happened. By this stage, I have to say, I was elated, because you really knew that people wanted to see the film and it was an amazing thing to be a part of. No one had to push it. It was going into the cinemas and there was a real buzz about it, people saying, 'I can't wait to see that movie.'

At the after-party at the Galway Film Fleadh a man came up to me and said, 'You're the character with the disability in the movie, I didn't think there was any need for that.' I was in such a good mood until he said that; I didn't see why that had to happen. Granted, he might have been right. In fact, he was right, but I was so upset and I said to him, 'Why don't you have a look around the room, mate, and if you see anything at all you think might fit, shove it up your hole.'

We were supposed to go to a big film festival next in the US, but funnily enough that didn't happen after my name went forward. Turns out the lad I'd told to ram something up his ass was involved with the US festival and didn't want me at it.

When the film went to series I thought this is it, my character was such a one-trick pony in the film, a panto villain. He's the guy who wakes up, has no drugs, tries to shoot people with a nail gun and goes to jail. Then I get a call from the director, Peter, he's recast me as a schoolteacher. Overnight I went from being a drug dealer to a schoolteacher in a brand-new iteration of the show. Playing the schoolteacher, it's the height of irony considering I never finished school and tortured schoolteachers and myself so much. As I'm writing this, I'm off now to film series four and I'm so happy to still be involved in it all these years later.

It's been a big part of my life, this show. It's gas, when I'm walking down the street, people recognize me from two different things. Young people go, 'Are you the guy from *Young Offenders*?' and older people go, 'Oh, would you not bring back that hidden camera thing again?' So you can tell people's ages from how they recognize you, which is kind of nice, it gives you a feel that there's a bit of longevity in the career. You think, 'I must be doing something right if I've lasted, what, over twenty years in this game?'

Acting is a great job but again, it's a part-time job. You always know: I'm not gonna become a full-time actor, it's never gonna happen. This gig, much as I love it, only comes around once every couple of years. Every couple of years I've to grow a moustache, grow my hair and be physically uncomfortable with myself for a while.

Sometimes I say to myself, *You love acting but what has it really brought to your life?* You think acting is going to be this glamorous business, where you're swanning around in big cars or sitting in a fancy trailer. It's not. As often as not, you're sitting in a draughty GAA hall somewhere. Maybe you film a paragraph a day on a twelve-hour shoot. But most of the time you spend eating sandwiches, cheesecake and biscuits.

So, twenty-four years after acting school, I can honestly, definitively say acting has brought fatness into my life.

As much as I dislike and give out about comedy, comedy gave me money and options. It gave me travel and a place to live. It paid my bills and bought me motorbikes.

As much as I love acting, it's given me next to nothing, apart from a bigger belt.

21.
Stage fright and racing bikes

As good as things were going with stand-up, I was wracked with stage fright, wracked with the dread of getting on stage. The torture I was putting myself through was getting worse. Even if the audience were obviously loving it, on their feet giving standing ovations, I'd still be thinking about how I screwed up the delivery on this line or didn't tell that story the way I had wanted to.

It could have been better. No matter how good it was, it could have been better.

The gigs were getting bigger and as they got bigger so did the pressure I put on myself. Other comics would tell me it was the opposite for them, that the more they did stand-up the easier it got, and the more popular they became the more enjoyable it was; they knew the audience were there to see them, they were on their side.

For me, it was the exact reverse. Soon as I realized the audience were there to see me and not the other four acts on the bill, I would take on all the responsibility for their weekends and their good times. It all just felt like such a massive weight on my shoulders: it's up to me now. If these people have a terrible time after working hard all week, it's me that's ruined their weekend. And if I let them down, I've let myself down.

I understood stand-up was a great way to make a living. And I understood that the hours were great and loads of people would swap to have the life I was living. But at the end of the day, I didn't enjoy the process of gigging. What I enjoyed was walking off the stage at the end. Instead of thinking, 'Isn't this great,' I spent all my time wishing there was something else I could do and every year the pressure was getting heavier and heavier and harder and harder.

Sometimes I'd go away with other comics to Montreal or Dubai, and they'd all be excited and looking forward to their gigs. Afterwards they'd be high on adrenaline and want to go have a few drinks. But I never wanted to do any of that, I wanted to isolate myself, just sit down, watch TV, try and get my head back and once I'd done that, start worrying about the next gig. That's all that really happened to me – get through that night and then wake up and start all over again. It felt like self-abuse in a way.

With every new show you'd get to the stage where you could relax a bit because you knew it was working and it was bulletproof. But by that point you'd done the show so many times you had to wrap it up. That's the inevitable, horrible reality of doing stand-up: by the time you do your last night on a tour, and the show is just about perfect, the way it should be, you've done it so many times no one wants to see it again. Every stand-up will tell you that.

What helped was racing motorbikes. That feeling I'd first had as a kid, being able to ride off anywhere, dreaming of

Evel Knievel. It was an escape from feeling out of synch with everything around me, the whole world telling me everything was going great for me when my reality was I was wracked with stress and anxiety. So it was just great to go out and race a motorbike on the weekends. No matter what was going on, there was motorbike racing to look forward to.

Most of the money I was making was going on motorbikes; it became like a drug, and I mean an actual drug. I knew it at the time, but I didn't care because I was living for the weekend, living for that feeling of getting to the starting line of a motorcycle race. There's no feeling in the world like it, no feeling in the world is like a motorbike race. Steve McQueen once said, 'Racing is life and everything else is just hanging around.' And it's so true.

I know I'll never reach those heights again. Getting out there on a Saturday or a Sunday, sitting on the starting line and watching those lights go red. Bricking myself that I wouldn't even get around the first corner in one piece.

If you want to really enjoy life on a Monday morning, put yourself through a near-death experience on a Sunday evening. If you spend your weekend wondering what shape your body's going to be in on a Monday morning, you can rest assured that you're living your life.

My thinking is: don't put a perfectly preserved body into the ground. You wasted it. Put a shagged-down piece of shite into the ground, make sure you've used every last bit of it. Don't just sit in a pub wrecking it. Everything that's used well ends up wrecked, and your body shouldn't be any different. I wouldn't swap my limps and bumps and broken bones for anything.

Those were the best days ever, that beautiful danger of racing. There's nothing else in the world that can give you that, where all you can think about is the ten yards in front of your face, or that one second you are away from crashing into somebody else. It's the best sport in the world, but if somebody came up with it today it'd never, ever be legalized.

'What? You want to stick an engine between your legs and fly up the road in traffic? Are you insane?'

Madder still, sticking an engine between your legs and shooting up a road racing thirty other lads with engines between their legs?

But it's absolutely brilliant, the most underrated sport in the world. The lads doing it now, they're the last gladiators. They might look like weird jockeys in leather but they're doing stuff that nobody else would do.

Racing motorcycles is the most amazing thing I've ever done but it tortured me. Because of racing my body will never work the way it's supposed to again. I've had bones sticking out of my shoulder and torn rotator cuffs. I've had my ankle operated on four times and my knee taken apart to put parts of it into my ankle. The other knee I've smashed up and I've broken my left shoulder. I'm deaf as a post from all the wind-noise and I've had several concussions.

But I can truthfully say, it was worth every injury and I would not change a single day. When I won the Leinster 100 Supertwins at Mondello Park in 2011 it was the best day of my life. I remember sitting in the van and crying the whole way home, tears running down my face.

You decide to get into racing the same way you decide to get into heroin: you start with the soft stuff and work your way up. Nobody says *I'm gonna get into heroin*; they say, *I'm gonna go and have a pint*. Then they say, *Jesus, d'you know what might be nice with this? Hash*. Sooner or later, they try a magic mushroom and then they do some cocaine until one day they're getting into heroin.

Racing is the heroin of motorcycles, except heroin's probably better for you. It's definitely cheaper. But the rush of racing motorbikes – it's the beautiful danger that feeds your soul. You're just completely caught in the moment. People meditate, or listen to chimes, or stick their head up their ass, or walk up mountains. Why bother? Just get on a bike and go into town. It really is that easy.

When you're racing you sit at the start line and there's all these engines revving and revving and revving and revving, and everyone's looking, waiting for the flag to drop. They say when the flag drops, the bullshit stops. As soon as you move off the line, you could be paralysed, broken up, have a broken bone, have a concussion, or be dead within fifteen minutes. But if you make it and you've a trophy after it, there's no feeling in the world like it.

I retired from racing in 2014 because some fella drove into me and nearly killed me stone dead in Spain. I'd just finished the Killalane Road Races in north Dublin and gone up to the Ulster Grand Prix outside Belfast and then I went off to do a race in Spain. The body was starting to feel it, but I still wanted to try and get an international licence to do the Manx Grand Prix on the Isle of Man. It's the exact same track as the famous TT races, but one step down. To get the international licence your times had to be good enough, you had to earn your stripes and attain a certain speed consistency. So, I went to Almería to do a pre-season race. Flying around a corner I got hit and thrown off my bike. Apparently, I went to take a left-hand turn as fast as I could and another racer thought he could pull up on my inside and he T-boned me completely at about a hundred miles an hour.

When the paramedics were cutting me out of my suit, I was very confused; I kept asking them what tattoo I was getting. It's hard for me to remember that day, all my memories are in the wrong order. At about 3am I woke up to find myself standing naked in the middle of the room in complete darkness. Looking back, I probably should have still been under medical supervision and not on my own.

The next morning I rented a car and drove from Almería to Málaga so I could fly home early. At the airport I called my friend Pat Duffy and told him, 'I have to come home – I had a crash, I'm okay but it was a big one and the bike is in rag order.' As I was talking to him I went over to sit on a bench. Only it wasn't a bench; it was a Lancôme display in duty-free and I fell right through it, smashing everything. I made such a mess they had to cordon off the entire area. It turned out it was just another concussion but a pretty severe one.

I went out on the bike one more time. I was in Mondello Park racing around the corners as fast as I could when I saw a guy coming up underneath me. Normally, I would just lean over – *if he crashes into me, who cares, he won't try that again* – but I chickened out. I stood the bike up and let him go past me. That was the moment I knew I didn't have what it took any more.

With racing if you think you're going to get hurt, you're going to get hurt. That day I realized I was human, and I didn't like it, and because of that I wasn't lost in the natural flow of racing, I was too self-conscious. My international licence arrived some time later and if I'd used it I might have crashed and died. Thinking I've dodged that fate is the only thing that comforts me about having to give up. Although, it's not true to say I gave up – nobody gives up racing, it's racing that gives up on you.

*

Racing bikes there does come a point with it when you know you have to stop. It's when you realize you're frightened. As soon as you go out and you're afraid, or you think that you're not going to try and make a pass, or you think that you're not going to be able to brake as late as you need to, you're in someone's way. Someone more competitive than you deserves your spot on the grid.

Much like stand-up. The day you're on that stage and you don't feel competitive is the day you're in somebody else's way. And if you've been getting on a stage for five or six years and you've never ripped up the room, never blown the roof off – which is what every stand-up should be aiming for – you're in the way. If you're not leaving people in actual physical pain from laughing, you're in the way.

But I'm making them think, you might say. Grand, but that's not stand-up. Don't make 'em think, make 'em LAUGH. Give them an experience so that when they leave that room their whole body has had a workout.

The best way to find out how little you have to say to the world is to start getting paid to talk for a living; that's when you'll realize how uninteresting you really are as a human being. How uninteresting all human beings are. And this thing about stand-up being a great art form? All right, sometimes, *sometimes* it feels like that, but most of the time you're lion-taming.

Your microphone is a whip and the lions are all drunk. Your job is to try and dominate a room and distract people the same way you do with kids, waving your arms around and saying funny stuff for an hour and twenty minutes. Keep them completely distracted. Make them forget what's in the real world. It's not your job to make people think. They can think completely independently without you.

When you're funny for money, your *job* is to make 'em laugh. And then get in the car, get the hell home and pay your rent.

I don't want to be an old stand-up. I don't want to be the aul lad going around delivering jokes, sitting in dressing-rooms listening to my own support act tell gags, living on petrol station sandwiches.*

You only get one chance to be new in this business and at a certain point you become a falling star. I had my chance to be new and now I'm over twenty years down the road. You don't get two chances to be new and I'm not going to England, I'd rather stick my head up my own arse and scream *Who turned the lights out?* than go to England or Australia or America.

So, what am I going to do? I still want to talk. Telling stories is still the only thing I know I'm good at. So when the radio job comes along it feels like the most obvious perfect jump for me. Why not jump on what is already a dying medium? Nobody suits a dying medium more than me.

I caught the fag end of terrestrial TV by the tail. It was just about to fall off the face of the earth when we made *Naked Camera*. Not long afterwards Netflix comes along with a sledgehammer and just destroys regional television. And now podcasts are doing the same to radio. So, it was a perfect time for me to get into radio, just as podcasts were starting to be big.

---

* Probably the best advice I've ever given anyone, it's the Rule of the Road, something you should all learn – when you're in a petrol station, never buy an unwrapped cake. I once saw a lad pick up a muffin and stick his nose in it and put it back down.

Don't get me wrong. I love podcasting as a format. Digital media has changed the broadcasting game, changed the nature of the conversation: someone asks you questions, and you can literally spend an hour answering them properly. And then you get to feel like, 'I've represented myself fairly.' Plus, you don't sit there pouring your heart out only for the host to cut in mid-flow to go to an ad break or say, *That's amazing. AND we're giving away a washing machine if you can tell us the capital of France. Is it Paris, Berlin or Madrid?*

A job in radio has a shelf life. It's a great job but every three months you're up for a review. Every three months your figures come in. Every three months over a space of a year if your figures go down three or four times in a row your job is in the toilet. They're not going to keep you on out of nostalgia. You're gone.

I will always be grateful to stand-up, though, because I owe it so much. Stand-up paid for all the great things that I've been able to do in my life. It paid for me to travel around the whole world. It paid my bills for years. And for all my giving out about it, when a stand-up show goes well, it's really enjoyable. But the pressure just knocked the fun out of it for me.

Whatever savings I had are gone, there's a decent pension pot but it's far from what it was. And soon I'll have two little cost centres to look after who'll be good for nothing for quite a while.

22.
Meet the parents 2

My first motorbike was a Suzuki Intruder. Sounds like a fella they'd make a true crime documentary about, doesn't it? The Suzuki Intruder.

At one point I'd two Vespas but I smashed up both. One of the Vespas I smashed into a Frenchman's car. The crash wasn't anyone's fault exactly, just one of those things. He was turning right at a junction in Fairview as I was coming up behind him, about to go straight through the junction. If he'd kept going nothing would have happened. But for some reason – some sort of reflex action when he spotted me coming up behind him – he hit the brakes so, instead of passing the rear of his car, I slammed straight into it. As I went up in the air I remember thinking, 'I better put my legs out to try and stop myself spinning.' And then I looked up and I could see the car. So, I was completely upside down, completely disorientated.

My mobile phone was in the top left-hand pocket of my jacket, and as I was spinning I could see the phone coming out of that pocket, passing by my head. They always say, before you die you'll see dead family members, or you'll meet the dogs you had to put down, or you'll see the tunnel of light. Or you'll have a moment where your whole life will flash before you and you'll wonder if you made the right decisions. All I thought was, *Well, that's my phone banjaxed.*

I landed on my back and I was lying there thinking, *I'm gone. I'm an absolute goner.* No one came near me when I was lying on the ground because I think they were all in shock and thought I was dead. When I stood up, this aul fella ran over to me and said, 'You should be dead, son. You should be dead.' Then I fell over and didn't stand up again until the fire brigade and the ambulance arrived. I could hear everyone talking about how I'd written off the Frenchman's car. *What about my scooter?*

When I met my birth parents they said to me, we thought you were dead. They had been talking about me – I don't know if they did that a lot, probably not – but one day my birth mother asked my birth father what he thought I was up to and he said, 'I think he's dead,' and she said, 'So do I.'

It turned out that they'd had that chat the same month the crash happened. Probably coincidental but a bit weird. It was a huge crash – car and scooter were both write-offs, and I landed on my back in the middle of the North Strand. But I walked out of the hospital two hours later with not one bruise on my body. No impact points, no pain, no cuts, no bruises. It was a real sliding doors moment because I could so easily have died.

When I started the search for my birth parents it was because I got sick. I got something called Reiter's syndrome, which you either get from food poisoning or because it's hereditary. I didn't know if I got it from a dodgy burger or a family I'd never met. I got in touch with the agency my parents had adopted me through, and they told me to write a letter to my birth parents. I wrote the letter all in one go and got it into the post in case I changed my mind. I included a photo of me on a motorbike. My hair was very short, bleached white like Eminem, and I was wearing a Daffy Duck T-shirt.

'You have to find them, you have to, have to. If you don't find them you're gonna make me feel like I failed you as a parent.'

This was my mother the whole time I was growing up.

'If you don't find them you're never gonna know anything about yourself.'

She had a point. We had all this lineage, all this clarity around the dog. I could go to them and say, where did the dog come from? Well, they'd say, Tara's dad was Tiger, who was your grandfather's dog and now Tara's our dog. Okay, so what about me? *You're adopted, we'll get to that another day.* The dogs' family history was a walk in the park but my lineage, where I came from, always felt very complicated.

When I had my first rescue dog, Lilo, I was looking at the poor little thing and I could empathize with what was going on for her. 'Don't worry, mate. I feel it. I know what you're going through, I know you're wondering how you got here.'

When the agency got back in touch they told me two things: that they were going to arrange a meeting with my birth parents (I'll call them 'Mary' and 'John'). And they told me that Mary didn't like comedians. That was one of the first things I heard back, *Mary doesn't like comedians.* I don't know why they told me that. I thought, *Well, great, that's a great start.*

The offices of the agency were on South Anne Street, right opposite the Gotham Café. For the first meeting they ask you to arrive at separate times so there's no awkward bumping into each other in the corridor. I got there just after them, pulled up on the bike outside Bruxelles, handy parking.

The facilitator told me that Mary was very emotional and might want to hug me and would that be all right? I was like, of course, she can do whatever she wants. The way I saw it at the time was: I was the one who'd requested the meeting, and they were the ones granting it, so I was always going to be fairly easy-going about what way it went.

She also told me that John was a bit stand-offish but not to worry, it didn't mean he didn't feel anything or was disconnected to the situation. He just didn't really know how to express himself.

But then we went into the room and the exact opposite happened. Mary sort of froze and stared at me and then John jumped to his feet and said, 'Can I give you a hug?' So it was really bizarre.

Eventually we relaxed a bit. We were just getting into it, starting to break ground, when, because it's Ireland, people started walking in going, 'D'you want tea? Does anybody want tea? TEA? Are you sure? *Is everything okay?*' You know that's the question they really want to ask but they have to work up to it.

They did that enough times that it became a running joke. Finally, a lad came in and turned on a Hoover and started cleaning up. Eventually he looked around, saw the three of us and was like 'Oh, sorry, bloody hell,' ran out and left the hoover there.

They told me it was 1970s Ireland and Mary's mother was just having none of it – letting the side down and all that. They were from wealthy enough families and it couldn't happen. Mary was sent off to Bessborough House, where she stayed for the full term of her pregnancy. Because her family had a bit of money, she didn't have it as bad as some of the other women there; if there's one thing the Catholic Church respects it's money.

Mary told me that when I was born they put her under enormous pressure to leave John's name off the birth certificate. The thinking was that a fella can make mistakes, and God forbid you'd ruin a man's life over an illegitimate child or whatever they called them, children born 'out of wedlock'. They pressured the girls and women to come up with fake names for the fathers of the children, some name that was a figment of their imagination, so that in the future people couldn't put two and two together and your man would be off the hook essentially. They think of everything, don't they? *Lock up the women, protect the men at all costs.*

One woman was so distressed she didn't know what to put down so she wrote 'Charlie Haughey'. Ever since I heard that story, I always think of this person that found their birth certificate and was just shaking their head thinking, *Him? THAT Charlie Haughey?* If you're roughly my age and you're adopted and you're out there thinking Charles Haughey's your birth father – no, he definitely is not! Your mother was put in a very bad position where she was really scared and worried and didn't know what to write. But it makes you think then how many fake dads are out there? Maybe loads of people said Charlie Haughey. Maybe that's why Charlie Haughey had such a bad reputation.

Since Mary and John were in a relationship, she put down John's full name and named me after him too, for good measure. Then, some time after I was adopted, they got married and had four more children.

I already knew all this, though. From a very early age my mother was always telling me, 'You have brothers, you have sisters out there, and one day you have to go and find them.' So she must have been in touch with the agency. Whether my mother was ringing the agency or they were ringing her, I don't know. Either way they probably shouldn't have been doing it but it was good I had the advance intel. Discovering it for the first time when I met them might have been a bit upsetting otherwise.

And then just as we arrived separately, we left separately, and I was standing by my motorbike on the phone to my girlfriend Elaine, telling her how it went, when they walked past me and we said hello. That was one of the strangest parts of the day – it was weird seeing them like that, seeing them in the wild, so to speak, just doing their thing. I'd never imagined them that way before. I'd never thought that they'd be normal. You think so much about your birth parents – who they might be, what they might be doing. I suppose in my head all my life they were like people you see on TV, characters in a story. You don't think of well-dressed middle-aged people just going about their business, walking down the street.

A short time after, I went to meet the whole family in the west of Ireland. When I got there I couldn't help thinking how different their life was to mine. You're kind of looking through this window at how your life might have been but wasn't. John and Mary's kids all finished school for a start. They went to boarding school and university and some of them were following John into the family profession. And I'm there telling jokes and hoping for the best.

There's no guidebooks on what to do when you meet your birth parents or your long-lost child. We were all just winging it. A few months later John and I flew to Tel Aviv, just the two of us, to watch Ireland play Israel, to try and get to know each other and do a bit of bonding. The whole thing went really well, but I'd just finished filming *Naked Camera* and a week after we came back it hit the screens and all of a sudden I was everywhere.

Only a week or two before, if I was down visiting them there might be some mild curiosity about who that stranger with them was, because it's a small town and everyone likes to know everything about you. But now it was different. 'Look, that's the "Dirty Aul Wan" over there talking to John and Mary, wonder what he wants?' After one of my visits John told me someone actually came up to him on the street and said, 'Jaysus, you're hanging around with some strange fucking people these days!'

At the time this was all happening, I was doing a lot of interviews, and had spoken to Ray D'Arcy about being adopted, so people started putting two and two together. Which was a pity because we were just getting to know each other and they would have preferred to have kept it all private for a while, break it to their friends and community on their own terms.

There were things I needed to know that only Mary and John could tell me.

Is there heart disease? No.

Is there cancer? No.

I've inherited really annoying stuff like tinnitus: in one of my ears it feels like there's a wave hitting it all the time. I went for a hearing test and you hold down a button when you hear a beep and it's all different tones. After I did that they came in and said we've bad news: your bad ear is pretty much deaf and you've tinnitus in the other one.

When I met my birth parents they were able to tell me, *Yup, that's definitely hereditary.*

And then I was sitting in their gaff one day and John was sitting next to me and he got this sneezing fit. The family were sitting around going, 'Oh, here we go,' and it was mad because that happens to me all the time. I said, 'I need you to tell this to people, tell people I'm not doing this to annoy them. I need you to write this down!'

A letter from my dad to say that it's a real thing and I'm not just being an annoying, sneezing-for-no-reason weirdo. So, sneezing fits and deafness and baldness run in the family but thankfully I've dodged that last one.

A lot of adopted people I've met really want to meet someone that resembles them. It wasn't a massive concern of mine, since growing up I really did look so much like my da. But then I met my birth family and oh my God but one of my birth sisters is the image and I mean the *image* of me. Or vice versa. Whatever way you put it we're so alike. It freaked us both out so much that for a good while we found it difficult to talk to each other, but we actually get on very well now.

I was always telling Kelly how much we looked alike, and she was curious to meet her, but then when she saw her at my mother's funeral she said, 'You don't look a bit alike, you look more like Arnold Schwarzenegger than you look like her!' So, I don't know, maybe it was just something she and I could see between us.

Looking alike isn't the only way you can resemble someone. There is an uncle who did go to college but then joined the merchant navy and is into motorbikes. He's great craic, a good head, real contrary, has a whole clatter of kids who think he's hilarious. Now he's in his seventies and still riding motorbikes all round the world. If I take after any of them it's probably him, isn't it?

What I can gather from what they told me is I was born in a hospital outside of Bessborough House, and I think there was a bit of panic involved in that; Mary really did not want to give birth in that place, and who can blame her. Again, I'm pretty sure that's true but it's difficult to confirm, these are things nobody wants to talk about.

There's still this missing bit, the six months I spent in Finglas after I left Bessborough House and before I got to Marino. No one seems to have documented that, I just kind of appeared in the Gallagher family. Then with my own parents there was a feeling that their inability to have children was something that carried a bit of tension and a bit of blame; it was shrouded in an uncomfortable mystery. There was never a deep conversation about it, and could you believe your parents anyway, whatever they told you?

Looking back has always been difficult because I have to look back through other people's eyes and it's uncomfortable – even writing this, it's not a nice thing to remind myself of. On a bad day I used to think of myself as this big mistake that caused all this pain from day one.

Sometimes I feel a bit like a rabbit that was pulled out of a hat by a magician, a weird magic trick that upsets people. My birthday every year is a difficult day for Mary and John because it reminds them of a traumatic time. So, if I ask a fairly standard question, such as, 'What time was I born?' what I'm actually doing is I'm bringing back really bad memories for the people who had to live through it, especially the people who had to give me away.

*

Twenty-something years on we're still trying to find where we belong in each other's lives. They do feel like family, but not close family. They're not my parents but they are also not *not* my parents. They're not my aunt and uncle but that's sort of where the boundaries of them are in my head. Having said that, I'm in touch with them a good bit and I'd only be in touch with my regular aunts and uncles if somebody died.

Sometimes my ma would tell me to ring my mother, meaning my birth mother, and I hated it; I wasn't angry or anything, it just always felt very weird and hit a nerve.

'You're my mother!'

Same thing when she'd say, 'Ring your father,' meaning my birth father. 'I can't ring my father,' I'd tell her. 'He's in Glasnevin cemetery.'

For me, when it comes down to it my family are the people I grew up with. If I hadn't been adopted, I might have had an easier life, but I know for sure I'd have nothing to write about. A regular life just couldn't have competed with the life I led with my parents in Dublin.

One of the first times Ray D'Arcy ever interviewed me I remember telling him that my birth mother had spent her pregnancy in Bessborough House. When she went into labour she was taken to the hospital, where I was born and then put under the care of an agency. I couldn't remember what it was called at the time – the Christian Home for Young Little Lads Who Shouldn't Be Alive or something like that. It became Cúnamh. That was the place on South Anne Street where I met Mary and John. It's closed now.

Ray was like, 'Bessborough what? Where?' So I told him, 'If you had a pregnancy, and you wanted to keep it to yourself, then you went and you stayed at this place, Bessborough House in Cork.'

Ray was clearly disappointed this had all come up just as the interview was ending. Not only had he never heard of Bessborough House, he certainly didn't know that it and some of the other so-called Mother and Baby Homes were open right into the 1990s.

The interview was a strange moment and is still vivid in my memory. I can even tell you that Ray was wearing a blue shirt with white spots on it that day. After that conversation with Ray, I started talking about my adoption a lot more, because very few people seemed to know much about what was going on in this Bessborough place and places like it. It was much like direct provision is now – people are aware that something isn't right, a couple of people try to make a fuss and raise some awareness, and finally the bubble bursts.

And when the Bessborough House bubble burst, it blew wide open. Suddenly, people who knew I was adopted my whole life turned around to me going, 'Are you all right?' And I'd go, 'Yeah, I'm all right. I'm the same today as I was yesterday.' After all, I reminded them, I wasn't there, I didn't remember any of it, I was born in a hospital. But people kept asking me, 'Are you all right? Bloody hell, you must be finding it very tough, all these stories.'

But I knew about these stories. I knew all about how pregnancies outside of marriage were used to keep women down in Irish society, how the church took children off their mothers and neglected, abused and even sold them. About decades of trauma heaped on to women and children by an institution that claimed to have some kind of moral authority but was committing all kinds of atrocities against the most vulnerable people. I read *The Light in the Window*, a book by a midwife who worked in Bessborough. I heard stories from Mary when I met her. For a lot of women there was nothing else you could do. That was 1970s Ireland.

Growing up in Dublin in the 1980s I watched the Magdalene women marching up Griffith Avenue on some feast day or other. And when we were teenagers a girl in the circle I hung out in disappeared for a few months and we all knew what had happened. It was just considered quite normal.

Down the years I've often thought about her child, wondering, 'Where's that kid now?' Because her child is a grown-up now. Still, it's just curiosity. It never seems like that big a tragedy when I think of that child – no more than I look at my own life and say it's a big tragedy.

My whole life I always have been and still am baffled by adopted people who say they can't get on with their lives because they were adopted. People who say, 'I don't know who I am, what my identity is, it affects everything I do.' It hasn't always been easy. Being adopted has caused me pain and anxiety over the years, but my identity? If I want to know my identity, I'll have a look at my passport.

I'm not trying to make light of it – clearly, it really does affect people – but I never really took it on unless I was already in a bad mood. Or when things weren't going great for me, I might think, 'Ah, yeah, typical, I was given away and now this crap.' And when life is going well? Funnily enough, being adopted has nothing to do with anything then. That's just the way things are.

A few years ago, I got grief online from an adoption group. In the *Irish Independent* I did an interview where I said I felt quite lucky in my life. I'd a bit of survivor guilt, knowing a lot of women and children didn't survive Bessborough

House and places like it or had come out very damaged, but overall life with all its ups and downs had been good. The Facebook group didn't like this at all. They said I'd been totally brainwashed and obviously didn't understand my trauma and how could I even look at my birth mother now after calling myself lucky.

To be honest I still don't understand the criticism. It was bizarre stuff. It seemed like they deliberately misunderstood what I was saying. How can there be a right and a wrong way to process the experiences in your life? Why do our experiences have to match up?

Over the years I've done some work with the International Adoption Agency. I like them, they're great craic, but sometimes I get a bit emotional talking to them. I was on a panel of adoptees one time. We were there to take questions from people who had adopted or wanted to adopt. A woman stood up to ask a question and immediately she started crying. Her daughter was from Vietnam and every night when the woman was putting her to bed the little girl would ask about her sister who lived in Vietnam.

As soon as I opened my mouth to reply I started blubbering as well, so then there were two of us at it. What I said to her was, 'Look, all this anguish you think she's feeling is in your head. I guarantee it. To your daughter this sister is her imaginary friend, I swear to God she's not hung up on this. She's only seven, so she's thinking *I've got a sister* one minute and thinking *I want to get ice cream* the next, whereas you're really beating yourself up and making yourself miserable over it.'

It was awful. I could hardly get the words out, I was crying so much. Finally, I was like, 'Will someone please give this woman a hug!'

23.
The art of conversation

There's the people who ring you for a chat – you know the sort? 'How're ya? Just ringing to say hello.'

Are you out of your mind? I have a life, man.

Now, when I say I have a life, what I mean is I like doing as little as possible. I've earned this time to do as little as possible and now you're ringing me and making me work at a phone call?

Male friends have always been a problem for me. All my close friends are still women. Ronnie and Ger, they're childhood friends of mine but we talk to each other every four months or so. To have male friends I have to do outreach. That's why I joined the RNLI and the Blood Bikes and why I've joined so many clubs over the years, scooter clubs and motor clubs. It's why I got into racing bikes and why I support Bohemians Football Club and go to the Dubs' games at Croke Park. That's the only interaction I really have with lads.

Eventually, of course, someone wants to meet you outside of the activity; they'll say something normal like, 'Hey, why don't we go down for a pint on Friday?' Or 'Hey, do you wanna hang out over the weekend, I only live down the road.'

Immediately I'm thinking, 'I need a new club.' Or, 'How do I bounce this joker away from me?'

It happens all the time and I really don't know why. Maybe it's because when I went to a girls' school, I learnt how to be friends with girls. I didn't have close friends that were boys in those formative years. For some reason I just trust women more, or I get on with women more, than I do with men. It might be a trauma response from being wrenched out of the girls' school and surrounded by lads. Maybe I never really got over it? I find conversations with women easier and less of a hassle.

That's not to say I'm a sparkling conversationalist. An ex-girlfriend of mine told me one time, 'You talk all the time, but you never say anything.'

'What do you mean?'

'It's all shite, you just talk shite.'

So, in a sort of inversion of normal logic, I set out to prove how right she was. We were in the car on our way into town, about a forty-five-minute drive, and I made it the whole way in without saying one single thing of significance. *See your man over there, where d'you think he got a jacket like that? That's unbelievable. Imagine buying a jacket like that. I wonder what age you get to when you think that kind of jacket would suit you. And this footbridge here that we're passing, I think that went up there in about the seventies. What do you reckon? . . .*

I droned on until we got to town and she was weeping with boredom. Still very proud of that!

See, I'm great at small talk. And I can do that very well at a motorbike rally or at a match. For instance, if you're in a Vespa Club with a lad you talk about the scooters – the colours, the paint jobs, the seats, the shiny bits, the engines, the events, the runs, the jackets, the patches, the helmets. Then you go to the bike club, you do it all again. It's just bigger. *Oh, look at that engine! Look at those wheels! Oh, they're so shiny. Where'd you get that? How long have you been in the club?*

I go to a Bohemians football match and talk about the results. *Last year we weren't great. Next year I hope we'll be better. Jaysus, I don't like the jersey this year. Do you like the jersey this year? Would you look at the head of your man over there, he's here all the time.*

No problem to me at all, I can do this for hours without breaking a sweat. Hours. I'm great at that.

I'm not the only fella who keeps conversation at this surface level. That is why when lads come home after being with their friends for four days and you ask them, 'How's Nick?' we don't know. 'Eh, he's grand, I think?' 'What's he working on now?' 'How would I know?'

I communicate with my male friends at a different frequency than I do with women. But it does have its limit. You do get to a point where you're the one just droning on like your man with the gas coming out of his nipples putting everyone to sleep.

My co-host on Nova, Jim, he's the king of small talk. Jim's a few years older than me so he's of the generation who say nothing about nothing. Jim is the guy who when I told him I was suicidal at the end of 2021 just said: 'Really? Okay. Listen, eh, I dunno what to tell you, man. Jesus Christ. That's terrible. Well, now look, do what you need to do. I'm not good at this.'

And then a few days later he goes: 'I'm only not saying

nothing 'cause I don't want to be going on about it.' Which is refreshingly normal.

Still, Jim was a big support when I got sick and went into St Pat's. It was Jim who kept the show on the road at Nova and he did a brilliant job.

24.
Losing my mind

You know the way if a man cuts his hand, or gets a pain in his flute, or gets a bad knee or a bad leg, he won't go to the GP until he's saved up a couple of other problems?

'My flute is burning when I pee and I can't hear properly. And the eye is a bit blurry and could you have a look at the elbow and the knee?'

We men tend to save up our problems so that instead of paying fifty-five quid to have one problem looked at, we can pay fifty-five quid for four or five, and we can justify the spend. Which is what I did when I went into St Pat's with depression, anxiety and childhood trauma. To get a bit of value for my money, I went in with a three for the price of one.

The only problem is I had to live through them all first. Anxiety and depression, they're like fish and chips, or a pint and a packet of crisps. They go together so well, they're the perfect couple. They're unbelievably complementary. So in synch with each other, like Kate Bush and Peter Gabriel in the music video for 'Don't Give Up', their arms wrapped around each other. They're the perfect dance partners and they will waltz you right into the grave. And then waltz off to the next poor bastard.

Depression tells you there's no point in getting out of bed and anxiety says the longer you stay in bed the worse things are going to get, so between them they will send you into a complete frenzy. Depression says you have to take a break and anxiety tells you if you take a break, you're doomed. So, there's no respite, you're trapped in a very well-rehearsed musical and in the last scene everybody's dead.

The whole way through the pandemic I never got Covid. Not one time. Not even a sniffle. But I did go mad. That's something I did do.

If I'd spoken up sooner and told people how I was feeling I wouldn't have got nearly as sick as I did. It's mad I let it go on so long, because I knew better – I've been sick loads of times before, but I was in a pattern where I thought, 'I'll take medication until I feel better and then I'll come off it. I might get a year out of that and then if I get bad again, I'll start the medication again.'

This was my pattern, over and over. But that's not getting better; that's just finding a comfortable degree of being mentally ill. What happens is you start thinking, 'This is okay, I suppose, everyone feels like this.' No, they bleedin' don't – not everyone gets up and has to battle with 'What's the point?' every day. Not everyone gets up and has to battle with 'Should I be alive?' every day. Not everyone gets up and feels guilty that they're allowed to take a breath.

Thinking and feeling like that all the time is just not reality. And that's what I was like when I thought I was feeling good!

By the time I started feeling really bad, all I wanted to do was get myself off the face of the earth.

So I left it till then to go and see a psychiatrist and I should have listened to him because he wanted me to go into St Pat's. But I was just so scared of the hospital; scared it was going to be like my childhood home in Clontarf, that I'd be surrounded by people who seemed to have literally lost their minds, and not only that, now I'd be one of them.

I resisted doing it for too long, even though I was getting progressively worse. The antidepressants I was on at the time were working so slowly I couldn't feel anything. So then the doctors had to give me sedatives, which meant I couldn't sleep or wake up properly, couldn't think fast on my feet. It was like I was slowly getting turned off, my battery was in the red all the time. I needed to go to hospital, but I wouldn't go. It was only that the people I was close to wouldn't take 'No' for an answer that I went in at all.

'You have to listen to the doctor. You need to go to hospital. You're in a really bad way. You're not getting better. Every time I see you, you've been worse. You just have to do it.'

If I had just followed my psychiatrist's advice sooner, I would have gotten better sooner than I did, but you can't get mentally ill and then look back and say, *I should've done this or that*. I only think that way now because I'm better; I couldn't think straight when I was sick because it's such a dark horrible place.

Now, most people don't go barmy. In fact, most people are sensitive about the whole thing. You go into St Pat's but you can't even say you went mad or you went loopy or you're a nutter or whatever because they don't want to hear it.

But I was all of those things, all of them, and I've no problem saying it whatsoever.

Some people there don't even like to be referred to as patients. In St Pat's you're called a service user.

Service user? Like I wouldn't even call myself a service user when I'm at the petrol station, it sounds so preposterous. Yes, I have served myself fuel and now I'm having a sausage roll and a bar of chocolate. But I'm not a service user, I'm a customer.

So, if I'm in an actual psychiatric hospital then I'm a nutter. Or I'm a patient. But I'm not a service user. That's pretty much how I see it.

I had no idea hospital was going to end up being what it actually was – a retreat. During Covid we weren't supposed to have anyone on the grounds of the hospital outside of the visiting area. But a friend was visiting me and we were bored and restless and I said, 'Come on, we'll just go out into the garden and have a walk around.'

We got caught by one of the nurses patrolling it and I asked him why it was off-limits to guests. He said the reason they were so vigilant was that recently there'd been a woman who used to walk into the hospital every day to enjoy the facilities. She just loved the hospital, so she'd come in and play bingo and go on to the wards and get some food. She liked the buzz of the place, got involved in the activities, spent time in the craft room, played a bit of pool, got into jewellery making. Then when she was thrown out she was devastated.

'I'm sorry, you'll have to leave, you're not sick.'

'So what? I like it here, I like it, it's my hobby.'

Can't say I blame the woman. St Pat's is the bee's knees. I loved it. I was there for eleven weeks. St Pat's is a place where you can turn off from the world and have people care for you. Even the food. I loved the food in there. Some people gave out about it, which I found really strange. I don't know what these lads were brought up eating – must have been fresh pheasant and venison every single day of their lives to be giving out about the food in there – because it was great.

In the hospital you have your own room and watch movies and go for walks and do normal, regular, decent things. And find yourself again. Before I went into St Pat's I was out in the world and I felt terrible and I wanted to kill myself. Inside St Pat's I was in this bubble and kept away from the world and after eleven weeks I didn't want to leave.

You can be sick for so, so long but then when you start to get better, it's unbelievable how quickly it can happen. It really feels unbelievable at the time because the liar in your head has been telling you every day, for so long, that you could never get better. 'What are you gonna do to get better? You think pills are gonna make me go away? You think I'm just gonna disappear overnight? I've always been here.' Like any bully, it is amazing how weak depression is when it's confronted.

Since I left St Pat's I just feel as if so much more is possible than I thought was possible before I went in. Before, life always felt very limited because I was always trying to protect myself. Worrying about how to get money, how to keep people at arm's length, taking chances that might kill me because I'd think, *Well, at least then it's over.*

I was terrified of anything that might be long and enduring, that would trap me, like relationships or babies. Anything like that I avoided like the plague. Even house shares were too much for me. Coming out and getting better I feel much more open to experiences and the things I used to love, like music and biking, I'm enjoying them now the same way I did when I first discovered them in the 90s. Even food tastes better. My belt is bursting off me and I don't mind.

All this healthy body, healthy mind is the biggest load of rubbish. I went into the mental hospital the fittest I have ever been, stronger than I've ever been, and I came out and now I'm fat. 'Tits McGee' this fella called me on the road the other day. When Conor McGregor had a go at me on Twitter last Christmas, he said, 'Get this lad a fucking bra, with his back bent like a prawn.'

So I know I've lost the run of myself physically to an extent, but I've never felt better mentally. Healthy body, healthy mind, it's not true. It might even be the other way around. A lot of people I know who go to the gym religiously are neurotic whackjobs and addictive in their behaviour. Here's another top tip I can give you (remember, the first is: *Persist with being idle until people give up on you*). Top tip number two: listen to Jinx Lennon's song 'Don't Lose a Stone for Christmas' and take his advice.

Like I can lose weight, anyone can. But can I ever make my ears level? No. And what does how you look have anything to do with anything really?

Since I left St Pat's I'm better, I'm in a good place, but I know it'll happen again. Absolutely. Oh, God knows how much fun that's going to be. There's no way I'm not going to get sick again. I'm certain of it. Recurrent depressive disorder is what it's called; the clue is in the name.

So, it'll come back, the black dog will come back, but now I have everything I need to chase it away again. It's like living in the Wild West back in the day and you find a bear in your kitchen eating all your food, so you get yourself a shotgun and a bear trap to keep him out. He's always going to come back and chance his arm but now you have the tools to beat the bear.

Even though I know I'll get sick again I also know I'll never get that sick again. When my depression comes back, I'll be straight on the phone, booking the psychiatrist, and I'll tell everyone around me and talk about it in work. It will never take me that long to get help again because I'll never do what I did before, which was to try and get better without help. I won't cover it up.

For me, resisting hospital for so long wasn't just about the fear of the hospital, it was also about the shame, the unbearable shame. I kept saying to my friends and family over and over, 'Everyone will find out. Everyone will find out. Everyone.'

'So, what? You'll have your life.'

But I didn't want my life if that was my life. The voice was telling me I would be better off dead than for everyone to know the state I was in. The liar wants you to cover it up, convinces you it's better to be dead than embarrassed or ashamed. Don't listen to it. Tell people, make a fuss, get help.

25.
The *Late Late*

Doing *The Late Late Show* itself was such a huge decision. The story was leaking out and I had so many people involved in the cover-up of having a mental breakdown; I was at the stage where I was going to have to tell people. And *The Late Late Show* was the one way I could tell people. Do it once, I thought, and then disappear and never speak about it again.

That was the plan. I didn't think anyone would really care about it that much and I could tell them all at the same time. So, *The Late Late Show* was the way to go, right? You say something on the *Late Late*, everyone knows about it, and then it goes away the next morning. Whenever I go on the *Late Late*, I'm never thinking I'm going to be the main event on it, that'll probably be Mary Robinson or Liam Neeson. You never know who is in the lottery with you that night.

I asked them could I do it, *Can I go on and tell this story?* Literally I said to the researcher, *I wanna tell the story once and this is the platform to do that on.*

I didn't wanna be known as the mental health guy. I've spent my life trying to make people laugh, talking about jokes. The last thing I wanted to be known for was being chronically depressed. But it backfired. Gloriously.

Kelly came in with me and so did Clint from Nova. I was on last, the act that's on while everyone's putting on their pyjamas and getting ready for bed.

After the interview I thought, *Well, that's the end of that then, I'm glad that's done and off my back*, and me, Kelly and Clint went for a couple of pints.

The next day it was the front page of every single newspaper in the country, I think, except for the *Irish Times*, because even if I spontaneously combusted, I wouldn't get into the *Irish Times*. I'm just not on the radar of anyone who works for, reads or has ever even read the *Irish Times*. But every other newspaper, it was front page news. Then I went on to my Instagram.

On Instagram there's a Primary Category for messages, a General Category and then an 'every other thing' category. I went on to the 'every other thing' box and there were thousands of messages, and I mean thousands. I started replying and replying and replying. After a couple of days, it was still in the newspapers and people were still coming up on the street to me and the Instagram messages kept coming and coming and coming. At one point I turned to Kelly and said, 'I just wish this would kind of go away now, didn't think it would be this big.'

Still, it kept growing and I can genuinely say, if I had known how big it was going to get before I did it, I wouldn't have done it. There's no way I would've done it, because I would've been too intimidated to think that there would be a reaction that big.

The thing is, I was still fragile. I hadn't done my year of firsts since I'd left hospital – you know, my first birthday, my first Christmas; my first anniversary of going in. I was still finding my way back in society. So replying to all those messages, I couldn't do it. I started scrolling just to see how many there were and if there was any way I could catch up. And it is no exaggeration at all to say there were tens of thousands of messages over the space of a week. Well, two tens of thousands.

Kelly just said, 'Put your phone down, this isn't getting you anywhere, you're just reading other people's suicide and mental health stories over and over and over again.'

Going back to being a functional human being was a terrifying thing. I was over a year out of hospital before I was able to say to someone, 'I'll do that for you.'

The thing is, in the hospital environment, the nurses are great, the environment's great, there are loads of activities and you're feeling really, really good. So, you put two and two together, and you think: 'good world' (hospital) and 'bad world' (outside hospital). Thinking, 'I've gotta go back into the bad world' was scary. I worried I wouldn't be able to look after myself. How would I go back to cooking for myself, transporting myself, being responsible for other people, keeping promises?

You don't plunge back into the 'real' world all at once. You get out of the hospital, and they make sure your pharmacy has all the medication and they still pay for it. They call you every single day to check in to make sure you are doing okay, that you're following a routine, that you're still aware that they're there. They keep your bed empty in the hospital so you can go back in at any stage because technically you're still under their care.

Just the fact that they're still looking after you, that's a huge safety blanket and if you add it all up, between the time I was in the hospital and the time they looked after me when I got out of hospital it was three months' solid care.

That home care package is so important and it's something that should also be available for people while they're sick and waiting to go into the hospital – calling you every day, checking in with you until they can get you into the hospital to observe you and really work out your medication. Because when they tell you you're going in, but not for a few weeks, and you've no one to contact but a psychiatrist who costs as much as a week in Lanzarote every time you see him – well, it's not very accessible unless you have money.

Getting sick is like the process of ageing happening at a rapid rate. You lose your physical health as your mind goes. You lose your ability to be involved in the things that you used to enjoy. Getting sick is about losing things.

When you're being discharged, they advise you not to go back to work, which I did not follow: I did go back to work. Because for me, the big thing I was terrified of losing was the radio job. The job at Nova was the only work I had in the world and I thought, 'If I don't have that, I don't have anything at all.' Losing the Nova job to me seemed worse than being dead, because at least I'd have died having a job. But if I lost the job while I was still alive it would just seem like the ultimate failure: 'Look at you, you couldn't even do that.'

Depression is such a bastard. You're saying to yourself all the time, 'You should be happy. Everything you have other people would give anything for. You have a car and great friends and a house and a great job.'

But then you turn it all back on yourself and beat yourself up thinking, 'Yeah, you have all that and you still can't be happy, you useless fuck. You're impossible to please. No matter what you have, you'll never be happy. You miserable, unsatisfiable, horrible bastard.'

It seemed to me if I could just hold on to Nova, I had something. But radio is a volatile business and you think, 'If I look vulnerable or if I look like I'm going to let the side down, they will find a way to get rid of me.' How is someone with mental illness supposed to be entertaining the world? Because when we sit in meetings, we'll say to each other: *The whole point of this show is to be able to tell people out there it's okay to wake up in the morning.* That's why we don't do news and we don't do fascism and we don't do heavy topics. And if we touch on those topics, it's to make light of them. We want our listeners to know that when you open your eyes and turn us on, we're there for four hours to let you know the world's actually not that bad. But if you are mentally ill and you think the world is that bad, you're useless in that situation. So you think they'll find a way to get rid of you.

This was my logic anyway. That was what was in my head. When it got to the point I had to go to hospital because I knew I wasn't going to make it otherwise, I figured they'd replace me. I thought, 'I'm gonna walk in here to Kevin, the managing director of Nova, and I'm gonna say to him, I have this problem and he's gonna say we have to replace you.' In my head this was a dead cert.

Then I walked in and said, 'I have to go to the hospital,' and he didn't even ask me why. He just said, 'No problem. We'll look after things; we have your back.' That was it. Then I told him it'll be four weeks and he goes, 'Whatever it takes.' This happened so many times over those three months and every single time it was, 'No problem, we'll look after things, we have your back.'

At this stage, poor Jim is having a nervous breakdown. It's true to say – 100 per cent – that when I was off the radio Jim was having a far more stressful time than I was. He's sworn to secrecy about where I am and he's getting grief from the listeners. 'What are you covering up? Did you sack him? You did, didn't you? You sacked him.' But they didn't sack me, they were being so loyal, looking after me, and still are.

Having the job to get back to, that was the rock my whole recovery was built on, how I was able to get back into society, how I was able to start again. 'I'll get up in the morning and I'll go in and I'll do the show.' And it was like a thermometer of how my mental health was going because I was back in trying to tell funny stories and maybe they weren't hitting the mark because I hadn't been on the radio for months and was so rusty. Then I'd crack a gag and get a reaction and laugh naturally and think, 'Oh yeah, there it is.'

That happens more and more, and my confidence is coming back – first thing every morning having fun with the team, having a laugh and taking that into the rest of the show, getting back to the ethos of the show: letting people know it's okay to get up in the morning. I'll never forget Jim saying to me before I went into hospital, 'You have to go away now and realize that for yourself, you don't believe it and you have to learn it again. So go, we got this.'

Everything I love about the job at Nova is the opposite of what stand-up is. I have a routine, somewhere to go every day. I work as part of a team and the work is collaborative. And let's face it, it's not lifting bricks – once my mouth keeps moving, I've a job. It's a very lucky, privileged position to be in.

The number one thing a radio show has to do to survive is to get bigger and grow, and I really want to be a part of that because they stood by me when they didn't have to. They had options; they had statements they could have talked me into putting out about stepping down from the gig, very easily they could have done that with one phone call. But they stuck by me and that's huge for me and that makes me enjoy the job even more.

And workwise, little did I know that when I did tell everyone, it would become the most profitable mental breakdown of all time, companies hiring me to talk to their staff and the radio figures going up. Bloody hell, I should have had a mental breakdown back in the day of *Naked Camera* – I'd have sold a million more tickets to the live shows.

I spend twenty-five years trying to be a comedian and then I become known as a depressed bastard and become popular for being mentally ill. There's a sort of an injustice to that but it's a funny injustice. It's an injustice that makes me feel good because I've beaten something that was torturing me.

26.
We will beat this thing

People say to me, 'Ah, but you're happy you went through the breakdown, I bet you appreciate life better now.' Yeah, I do. But I wish I didn't. I wish I didn't know or didn't understand the fight.

The best advice I can give anyone is not to take my advice because I'm not an expert. All I can do is tell people what I did and hope that that's in some way helpful.

I've said it already and it's something I'll keep repeating all the time about depression – and if you take anything at all from this, please take this: depression is just the most articulate liar, the single most articulate liar you will ever meet in your life. Depression's full-time job is to tell you how useless you are. To tell you why you shouldn't exist. To tell you that you are in everyone's way. To tell you that you're disappointing everyone you know, everyone you work with, everyone you hang out with and everyone you're related to.

It's a twenty-four-hour-a-day rolling news bulletin in your head that you cannot put on mute, lower down, or switch off. All its arguments are so well formed as to why you are a useless bastard and why you shouldn't be here. Listening to it – and you can't avoid listening to it because it's constant – is how you can get to the point where every cell in your body is trying to kill you.

Whenever you hear an argument that's counter to anything that this voice is telling you, you can't really believe it because you've already heard every possible argument that disproves it. Minute after minute after minute, hour after hour after hour, day after day after day, month after month after month. The negative is constantly reinforced. So, when someone goes, 'Oh, no, you're not that bad, you are a good guy, you deserve to be happy,' because you've been listening to Depression FM on a loop you have a list of 300 things that contradict that and are all completely accurate and truthful in your head.

The hardest thing to realize is that the voice in your head telling you you're useless isn't you. But it's so hard. It's so hard to say to yourself: 'That's not me talking, that's the illness talking.' Because depression says right back, 'No, no, this is you. This is you. I'm you and all I'm doing is telling you the truth. You know it.'

Getting to a point where you recognize that the voice is an illness and not you is the hardest thing, but once you do recognize it you'll probably, hopefully, look for help.

Your first port of call has to be your GP. Tell your GP what you're going through and have them refer you to a psychiatrist. The GP will give you a prescription that day to get you going. But you're still stuck with it for a while because nothing heals overnight. It'll be at least ten days to two weeks before you start noticing any change. And it takes four to six weeks for the drugs to fully kick in and make a meaningful impact.

Now, for a well brain two weeks feels like nothing. If you

were going on a holiday in two weeks' time you'd think, 'I can't believe it's so soon.' But if you're sick and someone says you'll start to feel better in two weeks' time it feels so far away. You think, 'I don't think I can make it two weeks, that feels like an eternity.'

Going to your GP is an important step, but what you really need to do is tell everyone you're not feeling well. Bite the bullet and say to your family and friends, 'I'm not well.' It's hard because it's not something we're trained to do. In Ireland, if you ask someone, 'How are you doing?' it doesn't mean how are you, it just means 'hello'. In fact, it's borderline rude to tell people that you're not well. 'Jaysus, I only asked him a simple question and he started going off on one, I don't know what's wrong with him.' Well, you'd know what's wrong with him if you'd just listened, wouldn't you!

Most people you tell won't know how to support you because no one has told them how, but you can figure it out together. My partner at the time, when I told her I was in a bad way, she listened to me and was like, 'Okay, what do we do? How can I help?'

That's the best thing to say to a person who's sick: 'I don't know but I'll find out. We'll get you a good psychiatrist. We'll find you the right medication. If none of these things work, we'll get you into a hospital.'

You don't have to lie or sugar-coat things with the sick person. It's not like if someone says, 'Do these jeans look good on me?' and you have to go to the positive. You can just say, 'Keep talking to me. We will beat this thing. I'll book your appointments, I'll talk to doctors, I'll go to the appointments with you. I'll keep you busy. You can ring me any time, night or day.' That's the best thing anyone can do for someone who's depressed.

27.

'Good good very good'

My ma's behaviour started to change after the *Late Late*. When I came home that night, she was in bed and there was a note left on the table for me that said, 'You are really good. So good. Good good very good.'

'Good good very good' is a phrase I've used for everything that I think is magnificent ever since. It was just so heartfelt. So inarticulate, but perfect for what had just happened. It's not even a sentence, but it just summed things up so well.

After the *Late Late* my ma started acting more human towards me. Anyone I ever went out with will tell you she could be a difficult woman to get to know. She wasn't the most accepting of partners coming into my life – I think she saw them as a threat – but she was all about Kelly, mad about her. A couple of times she said to me, 'You make sure you look after Kelly, the way you look after me.'

It was so out of character for my ma to say something like that. And then she started, like, asking me how I was feeling and things like, 'Are you sure you're all right?' and 'Are you sure you like your job?' And being very open – 'I care so much about you. I love you.' All this stuff that was very unusual for her.

It was like she was becoming a different person. She was getting ready. There may be no way somebody can predict their own death, but I think to some degree, people know when the body is about to give up on them and they're on the way out. So I think my mam was trying to assure herself that things were going to be all right after she was gone.

Ma died on the 5th of November, which I'll never forget: 'Remember, remember the 5th of November.' And like Guy Fawkes she went out with a bang.

When my da was dying I sat in the hospital for ten days and literally I only left to get food, go back to the room and eat it. One day I took a break, went home and went to sleep. I was running down the stairs to get back to the hospital when the phone rang and it was my uncle. 'I'm sorry to hear about your dad.' He had died in that tiny, tiny window.

When my ma collapsed and went into the hospital, straight away afterwards she seemed okay. She was chatting to me and Stacey up in her hospital room and had a bit of dinner. The plan was for her to get some sleep and we'd be back in the morning after her breakfast.

Seven am the next day Kelly and I took Kelly's dog out to Powerscourt for a run and had a lovely time. About 10am, as we're on the way back in the car, the phone rings and it's my ma's doctor from the hospital. He says, 'Hey, PJ, do you know your mother's condition this morning?' I said I didn't know anything about her condition but I was on my way in to see her. And he goes, 'Unfortunately your mother died ten minutes ago.'

Kelly pulled the car over and my phone rang again. It was Stacey. She'd just pulled up into the hospital car park and was worried because she'd missed a call from the doctor. I had to tell her over the phone what the doctor had just told me – that ma had woken up, eaten her breakfast and then lain back down and died.

Every year I got the same thing from my ma for Christmas: a bumper pack of Penney's socks and jocks – my year's supply. And no one gets more value out of a pair of jocks than me. Like, I can get fifteen years out of a pair of jocks. The elastic will pop, the pants will rip, the gusset will thin, but I will get value out of those jocks like no one else can get value out of those jocks.

I had a crash in Mondello Park one time wearing 650 euros' worth of leather trousers. I fell off the bike, slid down the track, the tarmac burnt right through the leather till my skin was exposed but the Penney's jocks protected my buttocks and I got out of that without a scratch or a bruise. A pair of one-euro Penney's jocks saved my arse, quite literally. So I have a loyalty to pants that most people wouldn't have, and me ma would kit me out every single year.

Christmas 2022 there was the wrapped-up version of a wheelie bin full of socks and underpants from my ma. Months in advance she'd asked Stacey to buy them for me so I'd have them at Christmas. If spending fifty quid on the ultimate amount of jocks for your forty-seven-year-old son is not a premonition of your impending end, nothing is.

I actually feel like I've betrayed her now, though, because I've since found the wonders of a good-fitting pair of pants. She'd be disgusted with me. SpongeBob PlaidPants was what I had been called for years because my pants were more like kilts than underpants. When I'd pull up my jeans it'd be a forty-second tuck to get them back down into the jeans so they wouldn't cut the balls off me for the rest of the day. Now I've found the grown-up pants the good-looking people wear and it's a life changer. But I'd never get a wheelie bin full of these because they cost a fortune.

A few years after my da died in 1999 my ma sold the house and moved down the road to the seafront in Clontarf. I can't say she was downsizing or even trying to make her life easier; the new house was almost as big as the old one and had previously been run as a B&B, so now she'd nine toilets to clean.

Most parents have a place they like to sit and in her house me ma had her armchair and everything revolved around that Mam chair. Whereas me da used to have his cans (you know: the magic can), his bit of chocolate and his bills hidden around the Dad chair, me ma had her medication and crackers for the dogs when they came in, and sweets for the kids.

We were cleaning out the chair after she died and we found mad stuff. Chopsticks from all the Chinese meals she ate because God forbid you'd throw out tiny pieces of wood. And we found a list that she'd made of her twelve brothers and sisters. On the list was their name, the year they were born and the year they died. And because my ma was the youngest, all the way down at the bottom she wrote her name, the year she was born (1939), then a dash for the year of death.

28.
Hells Angels

When I started to feel better after hospital, I had a totally new lease of life, to the point where I felt like a teenager again. I was throwing myself into things and saying weird stuff like, 'God, even the air smells different these days.'

I was so happy and more than one person told me, 'Uh, I don't know if you're doing well here.' Elaine said it to me, Kelly said it to me, and when a couple more people said to me, 'You're kinda high, maybe they've given you too much meds and you're in a manic episode,' it worried me because people who go into manic episodes have no idea they're going into a manic episode.

So I went into the doctor and I told him, 'I have a concern, I feel like I might be having a manic episode.' There's a checklist he starts to go through: *What is your spending like, are you gambling, are you partying a lot?* Questions like that. And the answer was, no, no, no. We came to the conclusion that I had arrived at a type of happiness I probably had never had before.

There were so many things I wanted to do for years and years, but I had convinced myself, *There's no time. You can't do these things. You can't spend that money. You can't just decide you want to do something, then go and do it. That's what crazy people do.* I was sitting on money that I'd convinced myself if I didn't have, I was going to die completely destitute on the side of the road. When I walked out of the doctor's office that day I said to myself, 'Actually, I am gonna do all those things.'

As I said already, bikes have gotten me through the hardest of times. When I was a little kid in a house full of alcoholics I could get on my BMX and get the hell out of there. When my dad died they gave me a bit of peace. And when I had no work and no money I put food in my mouth working as a courier.

After I stopped racing there was a bit of a vacuum. I've always wanted to be part of a motorcycle club. So I went out and did it. Now I'm like a kid who thinks all I need to be happy for the rest of my life is two bikes and a bag of jellies. No, two BMX bikes and a bag of jellies.

I started hanging around with the world's greatest and biggest motorcycle club, the Hells Angels. Why am I going to start anywhere else? I wanna go to the real club and hang out with men with leather waistcoats and badass attitudes and face tattoos who call each other 'brother' and slap each other around the back, and ride everywhere together and eat raw meat with their hands or whatever the hell they do. I wanna do that.

Turns out I'm probably not gonna be a part of it, but I'm gonna hang out with them for as long as they'll have me around.

It sounds ludicrous to a lot of people, but to me that's one of my great life progressions: hanging out with bikers. We go out and we listen to Ska music and we clap each other on the back and have a laugh, and we all dress like we're still fifteen wearing our Ska clothes and punk jackets and talk to each other. It's still 1994 and it's brilliant fun.

And I bought a Harley. I never thought I'd buy a Harley. I used to look at Harley-Davidsons and think they were just two-wheeled tractors for little old men or accountants who dress up on the weekends and think they're bikers, doing 130 miles a year.

And I love the attitude of the Hells Angels. Like you spell it with no apostrophe because, *It's you who miss it. We don't.* I love that. That's a world I'm so happy to be a part of now.

29.
Nippers

One of my biggest fears, always, was my ma dying. The way I've always looked at it is she was the one who took me in when no one else would. Our relationship was never straightforward, we didn't communicate very well, but she looked after me and I looked after her. The only way I could cope with the reality of her dying one day was to think, *Okay, it'll be a horrendous day but at least I won't belong to a family any more.* That was the one silver lining I could think of: *My lifetime quest to abandon all things family will finally come to fruition. Then I will separate entirely from all extended family, just separate myself and clear off into the wilderness.*

Well, that lasted three months and now there's two nippers on the way.

Kelly came down the stairs shaking, and I mean shaking.

'I don't wanna freak you out, but I have to tell you something.'

'What is it?'

'I just have to tell you something.'

'Tell me what it is!'

She was doing that thing people do where they just skate around the issue. Kelly had something in her hand but I thought it was a choc ice with all the chocolate eaten off of it. *What's so upsetting about delicious ice cream?* That's where my head was.

The ice cream was a pregnancy test and it was positive. At first, I clicked into survival mode: 'Okay, well, don't worry, the world won't end,' and off we went to bed. At night we like to listen to something to help us sleep, usually soothing sounds like whale songs, bubbling lava, snoring puppies, falling leaves, but that night Kelly fancied trying a new podcast of true-life stories. Unfortunately, the first story was about a man who had kids and it ruined his life and the second story was about a woman who kept having miscarriages.

By this point I'm having a full-on panic attack, sitting at the side of the bed, my head all arched back like a werewolf. This went on for hours and I just kept saying over and over that this was the end of the world, the worst thing that could ever, ever, ever, ever happen. And I don't know how she did it, but Kelly got me out of that state; chatting to me she somehow made it all right.

On the day of the ten-week scan I was feeling sick in my stomach because I'd demolished a Wow Burger and chips, a load of cake and any other bit of food I could get my greedy little hands on. We went into the room and the midwife did her business and handed us a copy of the scan.

'Did they tell you it was twins?'

'Oh my God. Oh my God. Oh my God. Oh my God. Oh my God. I can't believe it. I can't believe it.'

So, now Kelly's panicking and my pants are warm with fright. I thought I was going to piss them. For a good five minutes the two of us were just hanging on to each other saying, '*Oh my God,*' over and over until we kind of stumbled into some chairs. We calmed each other down saying, 'Don't worry, the world isn't going to end, it's not ideal,' and on and on until we got to, 'This is fantastic!' Honestly, we went through every feeling in the world all at once.

Kelly's a twin herself, so now she's over the moon. Suddenly we're hyper and excited and we just unload on a woman waiting for her appointment and she's laughing and congratulating us.

Kelly goes off for her blood test and I'm sitting there with the picture of the twins, still not feeling 100 per cent and needing a pint so bad. That's the first time in my life I would ever say I felt I *needed* a pint. The excitement is sort of wearing off and I'm getting a bit panicked again.

We head to the Sheds pub in Clontarf, and just as the pint arrives Kelly decides to Facetime her parents in Boston. Now, I've never met or even spoken to them, nothing; Kelly and I only met for the first time at the Dublin Pride Parade in June 2022, marching under the Bohs banner, and we're only together about ten months at this stage. To make matters worse, Kelly is brutal at delivering the news. 'Okay. So, I have some news and it's big news, but then there's also other news which is why I didn't tell you the first news. And the news is, well, it's big news.'

It's like the worst episode of *Dawson's Creek* ever. Bear in mind this is my first encounter with her family. All they know about me is I'm the man who goes to the same football club as Kelly, I had a mental breakdown and a row with Conor McGregor. They only know about the mental breakdown because they saw me on *The Late Late Show*. That's all, nothing else.

They took it all well but straight afterwards I started to

feel more and more sick. We went home to bed. I had a fever, shivering, the whole lot. Eventually I fell asleep and apparently, I had a proper fever dream. Kelly told me afterwards I kept saying that I was in England and shouting:

'I don't like it! I don't like England!'

She was trying to calm me down, saying, 'We're not in England, honey.' She calls me honey all the time like a proper little American aul one from *The Golden Girls*.

'The twins want to move to England!'

Kelly was stroking my arm saying, 'Don't worry, honey, nobody's moving to England.'

Then it progressed to me raving about there not being enough spaghetti in Ireland to feed the kids and it got to the point where Kelly was shaking me and saying she was ringing an ambulance. Still I'm raving, back and forth between the two: 'Why am I on a train? Is this England? The twins want spaghetti!'

A full case of the histrionics. It's probably not an accident that I ended up in showbiz.

30.
Home

So here I am, for the first time in my life, at the age of forty-eight, looking into a void that is going to be a family and not freaking out. And that is because I'm in a situation where I'm not going to let someone down by just being me.

When it comes to being a father soon, I've packed in the fever dreams, but I still have my wobbles. I'm worried because I have two dogs, and while one dog is as hard as one dog, two dogs is as hard as five dogs. It's not double the work, it's five times the work to have two dogs. It's probably the same with twins.

I'm really not looking forward to the shit. I love my dogs and I pick up their shit, but I can't say it's my favourite part of having a dog, so I'm not looking forward to two dirty nappies nine times a day.

What I do to reassure myself is I tell myself I'll still have my hobbies, that once I can separate myself now and again, I'll be fine.

People aren't helpful though. Now I don't mind slagging, I love slagging, it's how I communicate with everybody – I slag and I laugh and that's more or less my creative process. But what is it with people when you tell them there's a baby coming? 'Sure, what age are you? You'll be dead before they're born.'

Or it's all, 'You can say goodbye to any kind of social life, you'll never see the inside of a pub again.' And then I'm like, 'Well, as long as I can get out on the bike every now and then.' And they say, 'Oh, you'll never ride the bike again, that's the end of that for starters. You won't be out on your bike ever again. Those days are gone, that's all over that is and you're going to get fat. You'll have no energy to burn anything off.'

'But I wouldn't worry too much about that,' they say, 'no sleep and getting fat are the least of your worries. Wait until the kids are twenty and they're out creating madness in their lives and taking drugs and all.'

I swear to God, people seem to want to scare the life out of me the minute they hear the news.

Over the years I made jokes about never becoming a father. I was really public about it because it was my biggest fear for a long period of my life. Now I'm having two babies because I can't do anything by halves.

I know there are some people who think this crazy American came into my life and convinced me to have children, but it's just not the case. Like many things in life, perspective changes. After hospital, my perspective on life is totally different to what it had been for so long. Now, I'm no longer this person who has to have these hugely defined rules in order to cope with being alive. I'm no longer someone who has to know as much as is humanly possible about the future because otherwise it's a void and that void is the scariest and most horrendous place imaginable.

After about a year out of hospital I started to realize that I have never actually been able to control anything. Any control I thought I had was a delusion. My best shot is all I really have in this life. It's all anyone has. So I'm going to be a dad. Okay. People a lot thicker than me have done this, some total eejits have done it and they've been all right at it. Did you ever meet someone's da and think, 'That fella is the biggest gobshite I ever met – how are his kids so normal?' Well, if fellas like that can pull it off, maybe I can?

I've spent so much of my life not liking myself that the last thing I ever wanted to do was leave more people like me in the world when I was gone. I saw it as a social responsibility not to do that, and having kids just always felt like another opportunity to disappoint more people.

Everyone probably has impostor syndrome to some degree, but I always felt like I was not supposed to be here. That's why I always did charity work: trying to justify why someone like me gets to walk through the day and live a comfortable life when other people have shittier lives. I never felt I had anything to bring to the party, so I got busy volunteering with the Blood Bikes and the RNLI and doing charity gigs.

People would say, 'Oh, you're a great fella.'

I'm not a great fella. I was just trying to make myself feel better. Comedy felt like such a useless living but if I could do a gig where the money went to help someone who deserved it then it was worth it.

Maybe I've spent an entire life in some sort of level of depression; I probably have and just didn't know it. Now it's lifted I think maybe I can do this. I might get loads of it wrong, but I know I'm going to try my best.

I don't think what I'll be is an angry parent, someone who loses their head. I'll try to be encouraging, let them explore the world, work out who they are and get into whatever it is they want to. I'll be trying to get them on motorbikes and into football fields, but at the same time if they don't want to then grand, we'll find something they do want to do.

I definitely won't be a conservative dad. I'll always be the one that says, 'Don't worry too much about school and results.' I'm not saying I'll be walking around with a ten-year-old in a papoose, or wearing sandals to parent-teacher meetings, but I won't be a formal dad worried about keeping up appearances and all that rubbish.

What I am looking forward to is being an embarrassment to them. I enjoy being inappropriate, saying what I'm not supposed to say and telling stupid jokes, so I'll be working on my material every day. I never want to go on tour again, but I'm going to be working on the dad jokes, the fart jokes, the snot jokes and how to prank their ma when she gets home from work. I'm looking forward to that.

Part of being a comedian is going out and asking the world to give you all the hugs you never got as a kid. People say you're an attention seeker and I'm like, 'Yeah, I know! I never got any!' So I hope I can give them plenty of attention and affection and save them from a life in comedy.

My focus will be very much on them trying to enjoy their lives. I want them to know they can come to me and tell me their problems and I'll reassure them that whatever they've done or are worried about, it isn't the end of the world. I'm going to try my best to understand them. I know it's such a cop-out to say I'll do my best, but I will do my best.

In some ways the whole theme of this book is trying to find a place to call home. It's probably taken me this long because without realizing it, I was completely depressed a lot of the time. But this is a chance. This is the chance to open a door of a place, walk in and say, *Fucking hell, I'm home.*

Acknowledgements

Kelly Doolin, we are probably parents by now and I need you to know how important that is to me and how I hope I never let you down or ever let Milo and Stevie down. This is a ride I never thought I'd be on and it's a ride I couldn't be happier to be on. I love you.

Ash, you were with me when I got through the hardest part of my life, I might not be alive if it wasn't for you. I don't know how to thank you enough for that and I hope things between us aren't too bitter.

Elaine, you're still the greatest person I've ever met. I wouldn't have gotten to this point in my life without you and I can't imagine my life without you in it. I'm sorry if I ever let you down, you always deserved better than me, to be honest.

To Hells Angels Motorcycle Club, I owe you guys so much for tolerating me when I arrived at your doorstep one day. You are the greatest motorcycle club in the world. Thanks for letting me stick around and thanks for riding with me and my ma to Glasnevin Cemetery after her funeral. You guys are incredible.

Thanks to the 81 Support Club, the support club to the greatest motorcycle club in the world, you guys rock! Thanks too to the pit stop crew for letting me join them and reminding me what it's like to be a sixteen-year-old riding a scooter for the first time. There is no better feeling really; I appreciate all the work you guys put in.

To Una McKevitt, you are the reason this book happened.

I bottled it so many times. You kicked me up the arse and got me started again when I needed it the most. You're a great friend, a great writer, a great artist and I'd be lost without you.

To my sister, Stacey, you are the only person in the world, I think, who can fully identify with this story. I'm so sorry we weren't closer and I'm so happy that this book has been a process that's helped bring us together. As mad as it sounds – we're both in our forties now – I look forward to us getting to know each other even more.

To Radio Nova who handled the worst situation I could have ever been in, in the best way possible, you guys are amazing; Kevin and Clint, I'll be grateful for that for the rest of my life.

To Jim McCabe, who I wake up and see every single morning, what a pal you are, what a professional you are. What a great bloke you are. I'm so lucky I got to meet you. The last eight years of my professional life have been the best eight years of my professional life and I don't think they will ever be surpassed. These are the good old days, man. We're living the best job in the world and it's the best job because you're right there.

To St. Pat's Hospital, I just don't know where to start. You saved my life.

Noel Kennedy, the doctor, you saved my life.

Kelly, the nurse, and all the other nurses, you saved my life.

All the patients who tolerated me and gave me extra portions of food, you saved my life.

What an incredible place. Honest to God, I know it sounds mad, but I wish I could go in for a few weeks every year just to relive how good of a system you have going on in there.

To my dogs, Wendy and Stella, who are right here at my

feet right now, you are the most perfect companions, the most unquestioning loving beings that there are on the face of this earth. I love you both to pieces. Thanks for just being around.

To Stefanie Preissner, my best friend, you know how important to me you are. I don't think I need to say much more than that. I will see you soon and constantly.

To my birth parents, I'm so glad we met. I'm so glad we're working things out. I hope this book is okay with you and I hope we get to know each other even better.

To Pat Duffy, my silent mate in the background who's always there and who has never, ever, ever called me, not even one time, without offering to help me. That means an awful lot to me. We don't see enough of each other, bud. I will be in touch soon.

To Damien McEneff, the Lord Mayor of Conquer Hill, and Linda in the back lane. Damien you are, quite literally, the dad I never had; right up there in that back lane helping me build houses and calling me every name under the sun. Maybe you wish you weren't helping me, but you can't help yourself either. I owe you a pint.

To Christy Burke. Sound man. Sound, sound man. All my memories of you are great memories that'll never change.

To Bohemians Football Club, the greatest football club in the world, you made me love football again. You made me look forward to Friday nights again. You made me realize Dalymount Park is the most hallowed place on the planet. What an amazing experience it always is walking in there.

To all the fans of Bohemians, you mad, solid, crazy black-and-red bastards, I love you all. To Hughey, the biscuit man in Dalymount Park, keep the Jaffa Cakes coming, boss. What a legend you are.

To the fans of Dublin GAA and Maher's Pub. I grew up walking around those walls and, every summer in the car park, watching lads screaming and singing songs. The only criticism I have, lads, is we don't sing the same songs we used to. Maybe we can work on that.

To Nico from the chipper. I was left with you and your family in those babysitting days when you definitely had better things to do. Thanks for the chips, thanks for the love and thanks for your time.

To Jason Byrne, who got me into this crazy business in the first place, I don't know how to thank you for that. You definitely didn't need to do it. I don't know how many gigs I ran out of you on but fair play for tolerating me and fair play for still being a better friend to me than I've probably ever been to you.

To Bren Berry, a true showman, an absolute legend, a man who put on shows for me everywhere, put me in festivals everywhere. A fella who seemed to think that I was good long before I ever thought I was any good. What a great guy you are.

To Lisa Richards Agency, it's years and years we've been together and, at times, it's like a weird marriage but thanks for being there with me.

To Faith O'Leary at Lisa Richards Agency, thank you for thinking this book was a good idea from the very beginning.

To Patricia Deevy and everyone at Penguin, a huge thanks for having faith in the book and for making this whole process a fun one.

To Eric Lalor, you sound, sound brilliant bastard, you incredible comedian. It's been a long time since we toured together and it's a long time since I toured with a lot of people but you're the only one who still stays in touch. When another man has become worthless to you and you still hang around, that says a lot about a guy and it means a lot; it's not forgotten. You're looking great these days, too!

Ryan Tubridy and Ray D'Arcy, you both gave me a platform to tell my stories, long before anyone else did, over and over again. You've always been so good to me, Ryan. The phone call you made to me that Christmas after I was on, after the most horrible things had happened, is something that I'll never forget. You're a good guy, end of story. Same with you, Ray D'Arcy. I love the weird curiosity with which you've always approached my stories. Thank you, man.

To my friends from growing up, Mick Carey and Oran Foley. What can I say about you, lads? You're forever, forever gone and forever always present, past and beyond. You guys are always gonna be the number ones.

Ronnie Whelan. Ronnie Ken Whelan. Yep, that's how I'd write it. You are my oldest pal now. I hope I can be there for you always like you've always been there for me. We don't speak enough, but that's just growing up, that's just life. Maybe now I'm having kids, I can be more like you.

To Mary Tynan, ever since the 80s we've been weird together and connected one way or another. You're a fantasy creative person and you keep me connected to the best year of my youth.

Andy Matthews, you gave me my chance at radio, you absolute mad man, I love you to bits for that opportunity. Working for you was a riot and always a great experience. I love radio and it never would've happened if it wasn't for you.

To my great, wonderful, gorgeous pal Kellie Harrington, you Olympic champion in sport and you human champion in life. What a great person you are. You make me laugh every time I see you, every time I chat to you and every time you

ACKNOWLEDGEMENTS

ask me some weird, bizarre question on WhatsApp, such as 'What's the Bruce Springsteen song "I'm On Fire" all about?' I never knew it was that weird a song to be honest with you.

To John Teeling, you were the first positive male influence in my life. Thank you for showing me there's another way of looking at things and that there isn't always a reason to be afraid of or feel shit about everything. It's no wonder you are who you are.

Thank you so much to my parents, Helen and Sean. My Ma. My Da. It was a crazy ride, but I don't think many people could have done better than you in that weird situation that we were all in together. I hope you know that I love you always.

If I've gotten this far down the list and I haven't mentioned you, it was probably on purpose to be honest, so go fuck yourself.

Maybe it was a mistake and if it is a mistake, I'm sorry. But mostly, go fuck yourself.

And hey, kids, keep skipping school, it's poison; but take your vitamins.